Electrocardiography (ECG)

Auhors

Jean-Jacques Goy

Cantonal Hospital
Switzerland

Jean-Christophe Stauffer

Vaud University Hospital (CHUV)
Switzerland

Jürg Schlaepfer

Vaud University Hospital (CHUV)
Switzerland

&

Pierre Christeler

Hospital Area
Switzerland

CONTENTS

FOREWORD

Since its introduction to clinical medicine more than a century ago, the electrocardiogram (ECG) has evolved into one of the most important diagnostic tools for the clinician. Most cardiac pathologies have an electrocardiographic correlate, and even in non-cardiac conditions such as alterations of body temperature, the ECG gives clues to the diagnosis and severity of the disease.

The eBook by J.J. Goy and co-workers on ECG starts with a comprehensive overview of the basic principles with just enough depth to lift the reader above the crowd when it comes to understanding physics of electrocardiography. The subsequent chapters provide an approach to the analysis of the ECG. The most important sections follow with insight into conduction abnormalities, arrhythmia, and myocardial ischemia. The eBook is rounded up by chapters on long and short QT syndrome, and electrolyte abnormalities. In addition, the eBook is accompanied by a CD with 150 ECG tracings which are explained by animations.

I have been struck by the straightforward layout, the very clear format, and the abundant ECG tracings in this eBook. The diagnostic algorithms provided prove to be very useful in my daily work.

This makes this eBook very attractive for all levels of physicians and health-care professionals interested in ECG and it is a welcome addition to the medical literature. Congratulations to Professor Goy and coworkers on this important new eBook.

Mario Togni
University of Fribourg
1700 Fribourg
Switzerland

PREFACE

Historial Willem Eindhoven in Leiden was the first to record an electrocardiogramm (Figure below) in 1903. The subject would immerse each of their limbs into containers of salt solutions from which the ECG was recorded. He assigned the letters P, Q, R, S and T to the various deflections, naming of the waves in the ECG and described the electrocardiographic features of a number of cardiovascular disorders. In 1924, he was awarded the Nobel Prize in Medicine for his discovery.

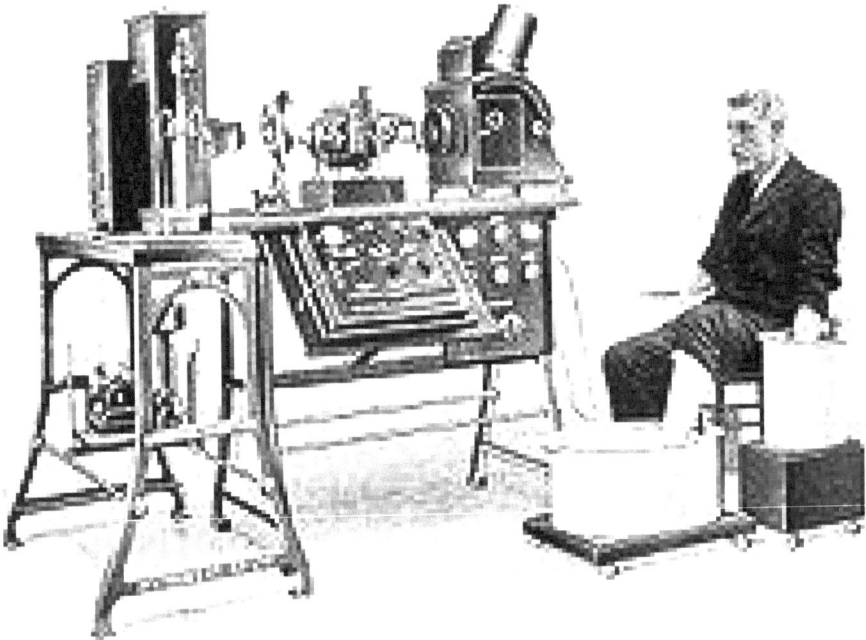

Photograph of a Complete Eindhoven Galvanometer, Showing The Manner in which the Limbs of the Subject are the Patient, Is into Contact with Three of the Four Electrode Immersion Jars in New Jersey, York

Though the basic principles of that era are still in use today, there have been many advances in electrocardiography over the years. The instrumentation, for example, has evolved from a cumbersome laboratory apparatus to compact electronic systems that often include computerized interpretation of the electrocardiogram.

With the need to stay as didactic as possible in mind, this eBook covers all aspects of electrocardiography in a detailed and clear fashion.

The eBook is aimed at the student who is starting out in electrocardiography, as well as the general practitioner who wishes to improve his or her knowledge and the specialist to use as an *aide mémoire*.

A large collection of ECG traces allows all readers to practise their ECG interpretation skills and test their level of competence.

Jean-Jacques Goy
Cantonal Hospital
Switzerland
E-mail: jjgoy@goyman.com

List of Contributors

Jean-Jacques Goy

Cantonal Hospital, Fribourg 1700, Switzerland

Jean-Christophe Stauffer

Vaud University Hospital (CHUV), Lausanne 1011, Switzerland

Jürg Schlaepfer

Vaud University Hospital (CHUV), Lausanne 1011, Switzerland

Pierre Christeler

Hospital Area, Morges1110, Switzerland

2

Send Orders of Reprints at reprints@benthamscience.net

CHAPTER 1

General Principles and Definitions

Abstract: In this chapter, we address the basic notions of electrophysiology required for the understanding of electrocardiography. Depolarization and repolarization of the cardiac fibers are described extensively. The action potential represents the transmembranar potential changes measured with 2 electrodes during cardiac fiber activation. The 4 phases of the action potential, related to sodium, calcium and potassium transmembranair flow are described. The electrocardiogram (ECG) is obtained by measuring electrical potential between various points of the body using a biomedical instrumentation amplifier. A lead records the electrical signals of the heart from a particular combination of recording electrodes which are placed at specific points on the patient's body. Cardiac activation is a depolarisation, with constant changes in direction and amplitude, recorded by the ECG. Four electrodes with conventional colours are placed on the patient's arms and legs to approximate the signals obtained with buckets of salt water. These 4 electrodes define 6 derivations: 3 bipolar, lead I records a dipole between the left and the right arm, lead II records a dipole between the right arm and the left leg and lead III records the dipole between the left arm and the left leg. There are 3 other unipolar derivations, called augmented (aVR, aVL, aVF), recording the same phenomenon but referenced to a zero reference called Wilson central terminal. To obtain standadized traces 6 unipolar electrodes are placed on the chest at a specific place. Because of their specific position each electrode explores a specific portion of the ventricles: V1 and V2 explore the right ventricle and the high septum, V3 the mid septum, V4 the low septal portion and the left ventricular apex. V5 and V6 explore the medium and lateral part of the left ventricle. Cardiac activation is the sum of all the phenomena of depolarisation and repolarisation of the atrium and the ventricles. The cardiac electrical activity arises from the sinus node, the physiological pacemaker, located at the junction of the superior vena cava and the right atrium; its activity is not visible on the ECG. The main electrical vector is directed from the sinus node towards the A-V node. The atrial activation turns into a P wave on the ECG. From the atrium to the ventricles the depolarisation uses specific conduction pathways. The A-V conduction is the PR or PQ interval. The ventricular activation follows the progression of the depolarisation along the His bundle and activates the ventricles sequentially. It is the QRS complex. The T wave represents ventricular repolarisation. Electrical axis of the P wave and QRS complex has to be calculated and is considered as normal between 0° and 90° for the P wave and between -30° to +90° for the QRS complex. In sinus rhythm, depolarisation is transmitted to the atrium and afterwards to the ventricle. On the surface ECG the consequences are a positive P wave in all derivations except aVR, a constant PR interval and a regular RR interval equal to the PP interval. At rest, the heart rate is around 60 bpm with a slight variation due to respiratory activity. A heart rate < 60 bpm is called bradycardia and a heart rate > 100 bpm is called tachycardia. With high heart rate the P waves are sometimes non visible because they are concealed in the preceding T wave.

Jean-Jacques Goy, Jean-Christophe Stauffer, Jürg Schlaepfer and Pierre Christeler

Keywords: Cellular depolarization, cellular repolarization, cardiac depolarization, cardiac repolarization, action potential, refractory periods, electrocardiographic electrodes, electrocardiographic derivations, cardiac activation, atrial depolarization, ventricular depolarization.

MYOCARDIAL DEPOLARISATION AND REPOLARISATION

Depolarisation

At rest, the cardiac fibre is "polarised", positively charged outside and negatively inside the fibre (Fig. **1** A). A stimulation (left of the figure) induces changes of the cellular membrane permeability with inversion of the electrical charges, which become positive inside the fibre and negative outside. Afterwards, this depolarisation propagates along the fibre (Fig. **1** B) until fully depolarised (Fig. **1** C). Transmission to the adjacent fibres uses the same mechanism. A vector represents the propagation of the depolarisation along the fibre with a direction from the negative to the positive.

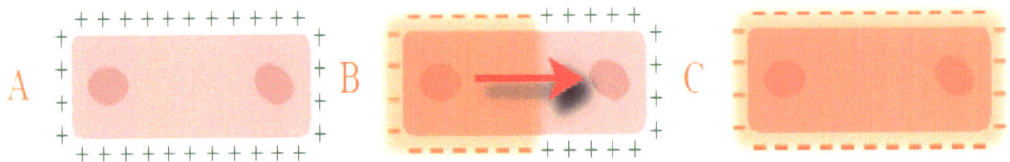

Figure 1: Depolarisation of the myocardial fibre.

Repolarisation

Fibre repolarisation wavefront follows the depolarisation wavefront: (Fig. **2** A) brings back the electrical charges to the resting state. Like the depolarisation wavefront, the repolarisation wavefront progresses along the fibre in the opposite direction (Fig. **2** B) or in the same direction (Fig. **2** C), with the same final result: a fibre positively charged outside and negatively inside (Fig. **2** D). The arrow which can also represent the repolarisation wavefront will have an opposite direction from the positive to negative. Depolarisation or repolarisation wavefronts are represented by a vector or arrow. The arrow representing depolarisation is positive at the tip and negative at rear. The inverse is true for the repolarisation wavefront: negative at the tip and positive at the rear. In summary the arrow shows the direction of propagation of the electrical wavefront: the depolarisation wavefront vector is negative at its origin whereas the repolarisation wavefront vector is positive.

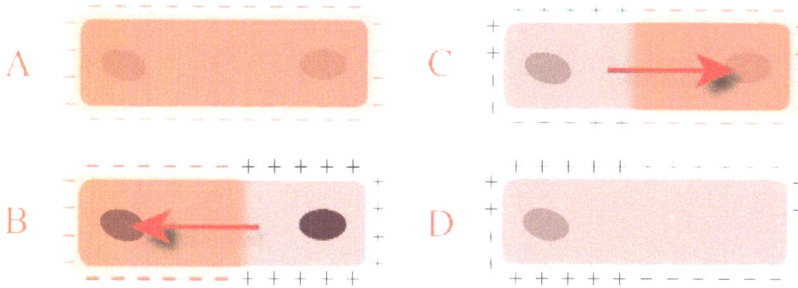

Figure 2: Repolarisation of the myocardial fibre.

Action Potential: Electrical Activity of the Cell

The action potential represents the transmembrane potential changes measured with 2 electrodes, (one intra and one extracellular) during cardiac fibre activation. The sequence of events that underlie the action potential are outlined below (Fig. **3**) [1].

The initial phase (or phase 0) is the depolarisation phase. Sodium channels open and Na enters the cell. The penetration of Na ions is important and fast. Transmembrane potential increases suddenly from -90 mV to +30 mV. Thus, phase 0 has a big amplitude, almost vertical.

Phase 1 is the beginning of repolarisation (which starts the recovery of the action potential to its resting value). Relatively fast with a low amplitude it is due to cell entrance of Cl.

In **phase 2**, Ca penetration maintains the action potential at a stable level for a relatively long time. It is the main determinant of the action potential duration.

In **phase 3**, Ca inflow decreases significantly, and is followed by a rapid and massive outflow of K which brings back the action potential to its resting value.

In **phase 4**, the metabolic cell activity of the membrane expulses the Na ions entered during phase 0, and in the same time brings back the potassium ions K at the end of the depolarisation. The ionic situation on both sides of the membrane is like before action potential declenchement.

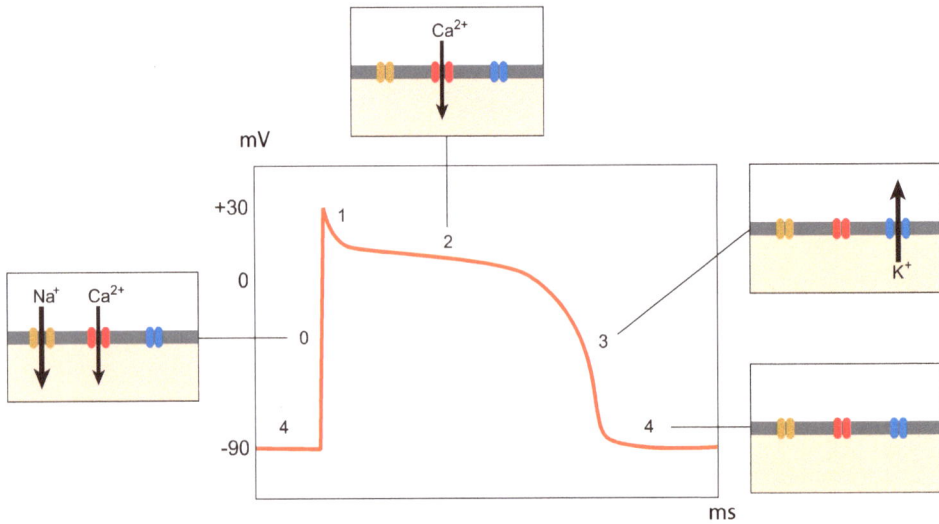

Figure 3: Action potential from the atrium, ventricles and His-Purkinje system.

These phenomena are in fact more complex, because 2 types of action potential exist: one from the atrium, ventricles and His-Purkinje system (Fig. **3**) and one from the sinus node and the A-V node (Fig. **4**) with the following different characteristics (important to understand the mechanism of arrhythmia):

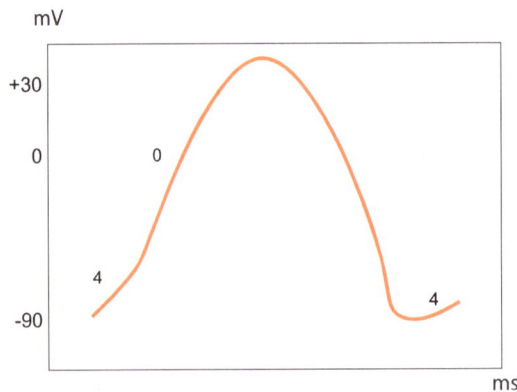

Figure 4: A-V node action potential.

1. Depolarisation wavefront related to slow influx of Ca++ ions. Phase 0 is slow as the conduction.

2. Less negative threshold (-50 mV).

3. The resting potential is oblique and not horizontal. A slow, progressive and spontaneous diastolic depolarisation is present and can provoke a depolarisation. This explains the automaticity of the sinus and A-V nodes. The rate of depolarisation from the sinus node is superior to the one from the A-V node the latter being active only when the sinus node fails: this is called nodal escape rhythm.

Refractory Periods

During the first 3 phases of repolarisation, the cell is in its "refractory period": in the first "absolute", the cell is completely non excitable (ST segment on the surface ECG). Before the end of phase 3 (T wave on the surface ECG) the refractoriness is "relative". During this period depolarisation induces a deformed action potential: phase 0 is weak, thus reducing the conduction velocity.

ECG RECORDING

An electrocardiogram is obtained by measuring electrical potential between various points of the body using a biomedical instrumentation amplifier. A lead records the electrical signals of the heart from a particular combination of recording electrodes, which are placed at specific points on the patient's body. Cardiac activation is a depolarisation, with constant changes in direction and amplitude, recorded by the ECG [2-4].

Baseline Recording [5]

When a depolarisation wavefront (or mean electrical vector) moves toward a positive electrode, it creates a positive deflection on the ECG in the corresponding lead. When a depolarisation wavefront (or mean electrical vector) moves away from a positive electrode, it creates a negative deflection on the ECG in the corresponding lead. When a depolarisation wavefront (or mean electrical vector) moves perpendicular to a positive electrode, it creates an equiphasic (or isoelectric) complex on the ECG. It will be positive as the depolarisation wavefront (or mean electrical vector) approaches, and then becomes negative as it passes by.

In A, the deflection is positive because the wavefront moves toward the electrode. In B it is negative because it moves away from the electrode. In C it is an equiphasic complex with a positive deflection as the depolarisation approaches and a negative deflection as the deflection passes by.

The signal morphology recorded by an electrode will depend on its position with the depolarisation wavefront axis and the direction of the depolarisation wavefront will move on this axis (the same being true for repolarisation wavefront); this is the fundamental principle of electroardiography (Fig. **5**).

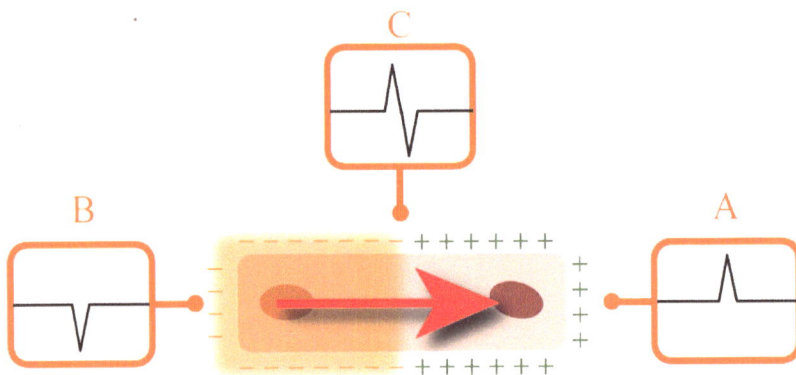

Figure 5: Signal morphology.

ELECTRODE POSITIONING

Limb Leads

Four electrodes with conventional colours (red, black, yellow and green) are placed on the patient's arms and legs to approximate the signals obtained with buckets of salt water. The yellow electrode is placed on the left arm, the red one on the right arm, the green one on the left leg and the black one on the right leg. The latter is mise earthed (Fig. **6**). These 4 electrodes define 6 derivations: 3 bipolar, (Fig. **6**) lead I records a dipole between the left and the right arm, lead II records a dipole between the right arm and the left leg and lead III records the dipole between the left arm and the left leg. There are 3 other unipolar derivations, called augmented (aVR, aVL, aVF), recording the same phenomenon but referenced to a zero reference called Wilson central terminal [6].

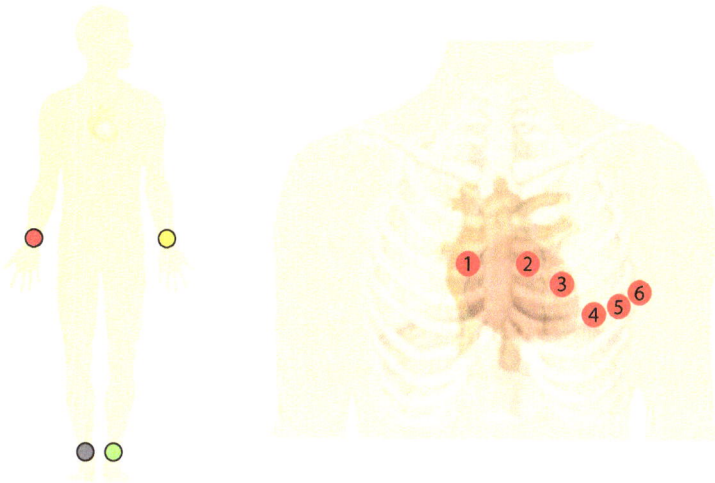

Figure 6: Electrodes placement.

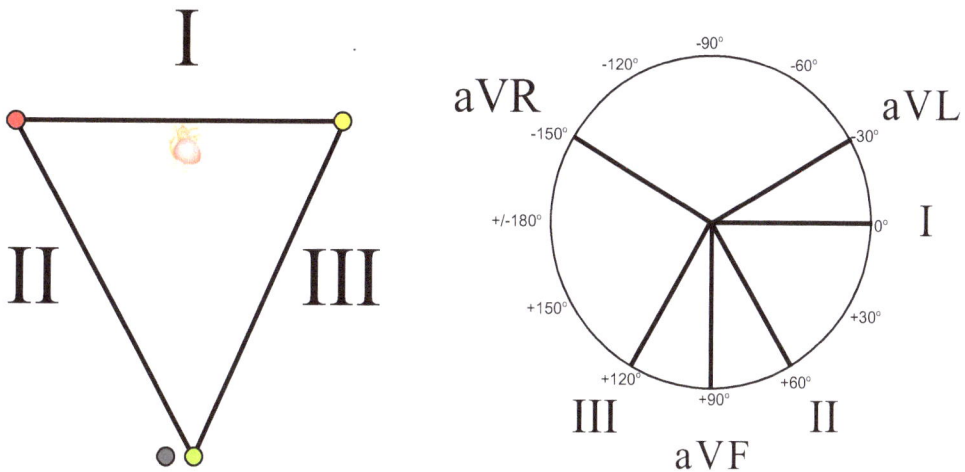

Figure 7: Limb leads with angles and directions.

These 6 leads (Fig. **7**) are in the same frontal plane. The 3 bipolar leads correspond to the sides of an equilateral triangle, and are separated by an angle of 60° and 30° from the unipolar leads. In practice the origin of the limb leads resumes, by convention, in one point (point zero), (in dashed line the negative segment of the lead and in full thickness the positive segment).

Precordial Leads

To obtain standadized traces 6 unipolar electrodes are placed on the chest at a specific place. V1 is placed in the 4 the intercostal space to the right of the sternum, V2 is placed in the fourth intercostal space to the left of the sternum, V3 is placed directly between leads V2 and V4, V4 is placed in the fifth intercostal space in the midclavicular line, V5 is placed horizontally with V4 in the anterior axillary line and V6 is placed horizontally with V4 and V5 in the midaxillary line (Fig. **6**).

Because of their specific position each electrode explores a specific portion of the ventricles: V1 and V2 explore the right ventricle and the high septum, V3 the mid septum, V4 the low septal portion and the left ventricular apex. V5 and V6 explore the medium and lateral part of the left ventricle.

In combining the frontal and horizontal planes most of the left ventricle is explored with the leads I, aVL, V5 and V6 and the inferior wall with the leads II, III and aVF [7].

CARDIAC ACTIVATION

Cardiac activation is the sum of all the phenomena of depolarisation and repolarisation of the atrium and the ventricles.

Atrial Activation

The cardiac electrical activity arises from the sinus node, the physiological pacemaker, located at the junction of the superior vena cava and the right atrium; its activity is not visible on the ECG. This activity is automatic with a resting action potential, which diminishes progressively (spontaneous diastolic depolarisation). When the threshold potential is reached an action potential is initiated. The main electrical vector is directed from the sinus node towards the A-V node, and spreads from the right atrium to the left atrium using specific conduction pathways (Fig. **8**) [8].

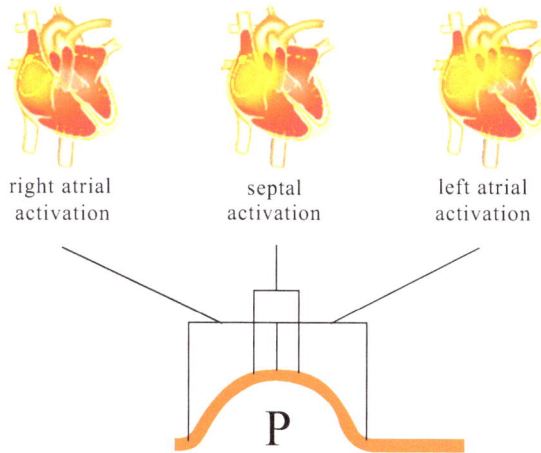

Figure 8: Atrial activation.

Electrocardiographic Consequences

The atrial activation turns into a P wave on the ECG. The initial part of the P wave corresponds to the right atrial depolarisation and the terminal part to the left atrial depolarisation. The P wave is usually positive in I, II, III, aVF, negative in aVR. Its axis is situated between 0 and +75° and its duration between 80 to 100 ms. A negative P wave in leads II, III and aVF, corresponds to a retrograde activation of the atrium (caudo-cranial) as seen in some supraventricular or ventricular arrhythmias (Fig. **9**). A negative P wave in I and aVL, means that the depolarisation comes from the left atrium to the right, in other words it is a left atrial rhythm (Fig. **10**). In addition to the axis, duration and amplitude of the P wave may change as shown in Fig. **11**. In 1, the P wave is normal (duration < 100 ms). In 2, left atrial hypertrophy or intra-atrial conduction disorder is present; in both situations the P wave is prolonged and doubled (duration > 100 ms). In 3, right atrial hypertrophy is present with increased amplitude of the P wave (> 2.5 mm in II and in III).

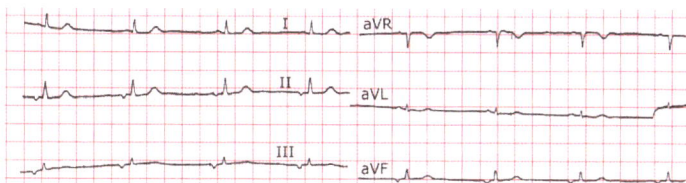

Figure 9: Right atrial inferior rhythm with negative P wave in II, III and aVF. This rhythm is sometimes called "coronary sinus rhythm".

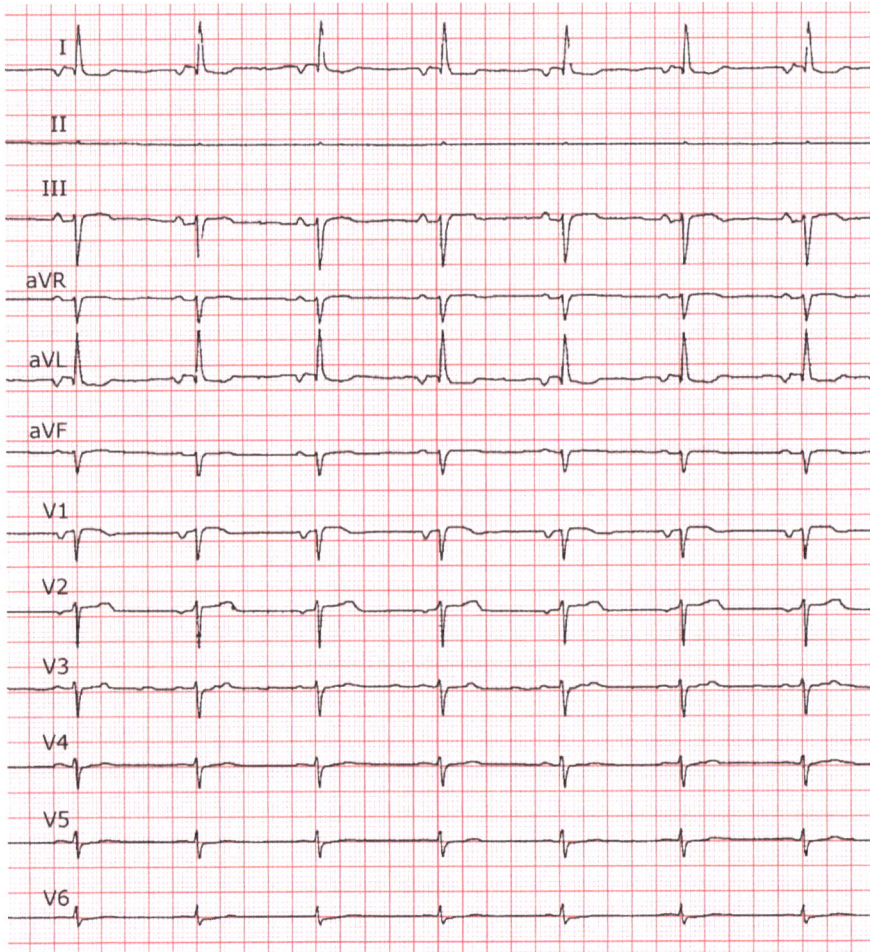

Figure 10: Left atrial rhythm with negative P wave in I and aVL.

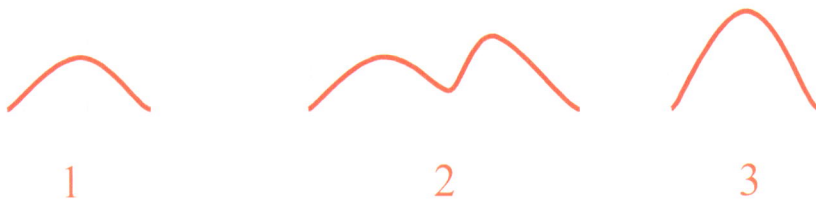

Figure 11: P wave abnormalities.

The A-V Conduction: PR or PQ Interval

From the atrium to the ventricles the depolarisation uses specific conduction pathways. The A-V node (Tawara node), is situated in the low right atrium and followed by the His bundle. The fibres of the Bundle of His allow electrical conduction to occur more easily and quickly than typical cardiac muscle. The His bundle's branches divide into 3 bundle branches: the right, left anterior and left posterior bundle branches (also called hemibranches) that run along the interventricular septum. The bundles give rise to thin filaments known as Purkinje fibres. The PR interval lasts 120 to 200 ms [9].

Electrocardiographic Consequences

Depolarisation of the A-V node and of the His bundle is not visible on the surface ECG; between the end of the P wave and the beginning of the QRS complex when the trace does not show elevation or depression.

Ventricular Activation: QRS Complex [10]

The ventricular activation follows the progression of the depolarisation along the His bundle and activates the ventricles sequentially. It starts at the mid portion of the left side of the septum, then progress to the right and forward: the resulting vector has the same orientation (Fig. **12**). In the derivation facing the left ventricle (I, aVL, V4 to V6) a small initial negative q wave, due to the septal depolarisation, a tall positive R wave corresponding to the left free wall activation and a small terminal s wave corresponding to left basal segment depolarisation, are visible on the trace.

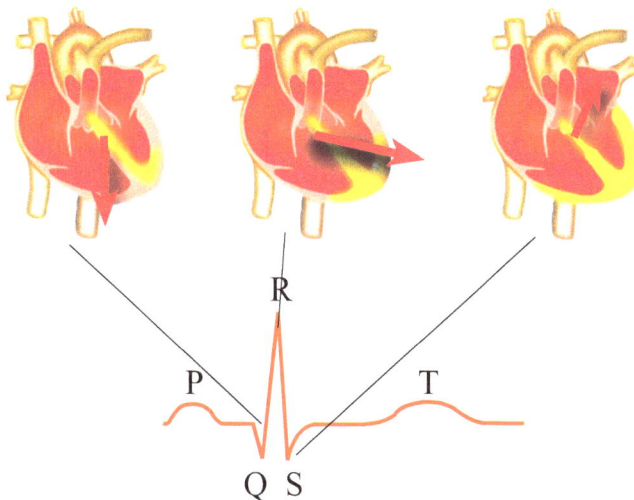

Figure 12: Ventricular activation.

The activation progresses to the ventricular sub-endocardium: the vector rotates left and behind until the complete ventricle is depolarized. The activation progresses in the apico-basal direction. At the end the most posterior zones of the ventricle and the septum are depolarized at the end.

Electrocardiographic Consequences

The electrical vector constantly changes in direction and amplitude. The consequence is a 3 phases ventriculogram, called QRS (in capitals or not depending on the size of the deflection). In some specific situations (Fig. **13**) the S wave is followed by a second positive deflection (rSR' appearance). The R wave can be absent leading to a ventriculogram with a single negative wave (QS aspect).

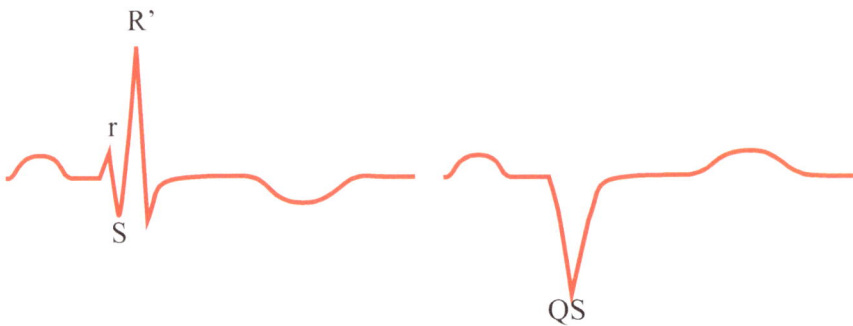

Figure 13: rSR' appearance of the QRS complex as in right bundle branch block and QS aspect as in left bundle branch block.

In the right precordial leads (V1 and V2) (Fig. **14**) the septal depolarisation is hidden in the initial r wave which should be > 0.5 mm in V1, > 1,5 mm in V2 and > 3 mm in V3, (when these values are not reached, the term "late progression of the R wave" is used). This depolarisation is followed by a deep S wave, called "miror image" of the R wave of the left precordial leads (V5, V6) and corresponding to left free wall activation. Transition usually occurs between V3 and V4. The term counterclockwise rotation is used when this transition occurs before V3 and clockwise when it occurs in V5 or V6. In V5 and V6, facing the left ventricle, the classical QRS appearance is found with a small q wave having an amplitude < 25 % of the corresponding R wave.

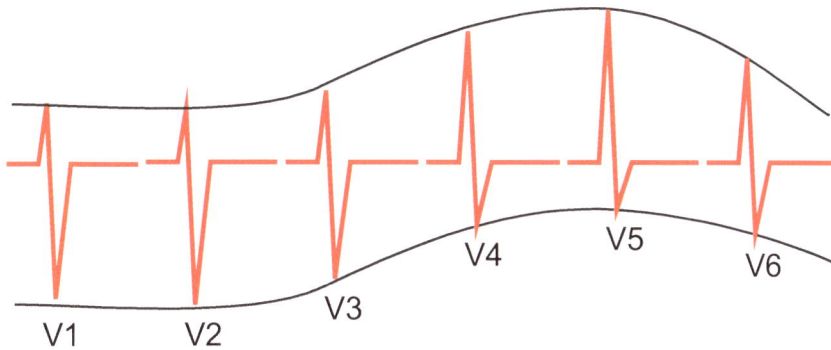

Figure 14: QRS appearance in the precordial leads.

ST Segment

The ST segment connects the QRS complex and the T wave between the end of the QRS complex (J point or ST junction). It starts at the J point (junction between the QRS complex and RT segment), ends at the beginning of the T wave and represents the superimposition of depolarisation and repolarisation. It is neutral with a maximal elevation < 1mm in the limb leads, < 2mm in the right precordial leads and < 1mm in the left precordial leads.

T Wave

This deflection represents ventricular repolarisation. Its frontal axis is identical to the QRS axis ± 15 degrees. The T wave is normally positive from V1 to V3, except in the children where it is negative. Persistence of this negativity in V1 and rarely in V2 in the adult is called "juvenile pattern". The ventricular mass interestsing depolarisation and repolarisation is the same; thus, T wave and QRS complex surfaces should be the same. Absence of this equivalence without cardiac pathology is called "non specific modifications of repolarisation".

QT Interval

The QT interval represents on an ECG the total time needed for the ventricles to depolarize and repolarize. The QT interval is measured from the beginning of the QRS complex to the end of the T wave. Normal values for the QT interval at 70 bpm should not exceed 400 ms. Its normal values are between 300 and 440 ms. The QT interval as well as the corrected QT interval are important in the diagnosis of long QT syndrome and short QT syndrome. The QT interval varies based on the heart rate, and various correction factors have been developed to correct the QT interval for the heart rate. For each increment of 10 bpm from 70 bpm, the value of the QT increases or decreases from 40 ms (for example at 80 bpm, QT ≤ 360 ms, at 60 bpm ≤ 440 ms, *etc.*). The most commonly used method for correcting the QT interval for rate is the Bazett formula (Fig. **15**). In clinical practice the QTc is abnormal if > 440 ms.

$$QTc = QTm / \sqrt{RR}$$

$$QTm => measured\ QT\ in\ ms$$
$$QTc => corrected\ QT\ in\ ms$$

$$unit: RR\ interval\ in\ seconds$$

Figure 15: Bazett formula.

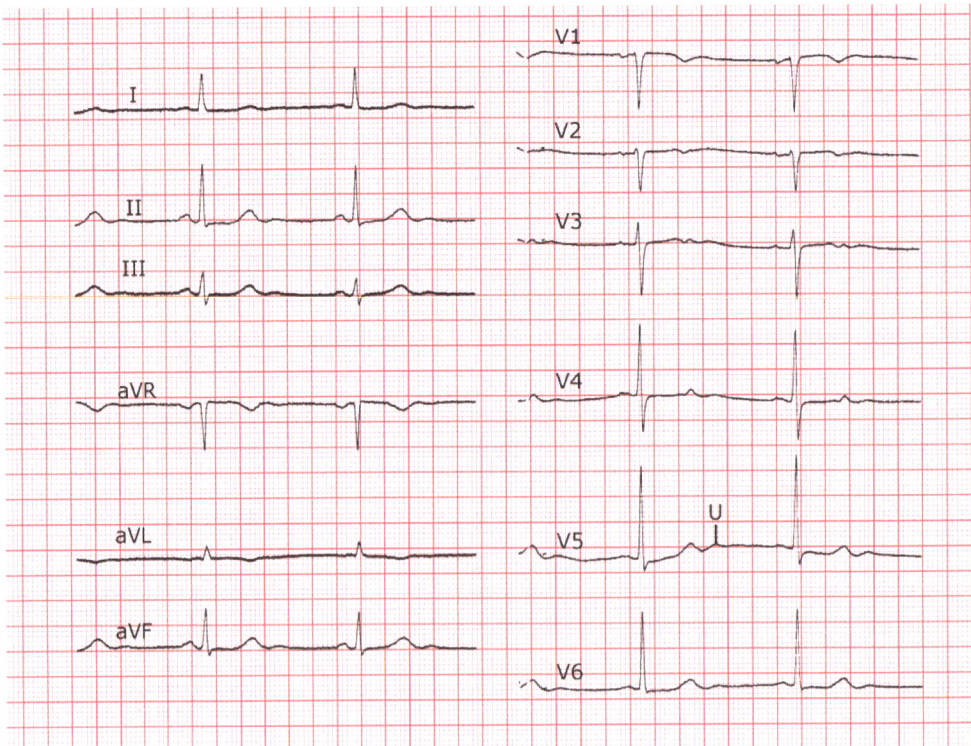

Figure 16: U waves visibles in the left precordial leads.

U Wave

The U wave is a positive wave following the T wave essentially visible in V2 and V3 with an amplitude < 2mm. It significance is still under discussion. It is either a prolonged repolarisation of the M cells of the Purkinje fibres or a mechanical effect due to myocardial relaxation. The U wave is positive in the following situations: normal subjects, bradycardia, ventricular hypertrophy, hypothyroidism, hypokalemia, hypocalcemia, hypomagnesemia and is negative in the following situation: myocardial ischemia and some cardiomyopathies involving the left ventricle (Fig. **16**).

CHRONOLOGY OF THE CARDIAC ACTIVATION

The P, QRS and T waves are only the projection of the electrical vector, which may have a completely different direction from the axis where it projects. In some leads this projection can equal 0, reducing the duration of this wave. Thus, measurements of any ECG interval must be made in the leads where it is the longest [11].

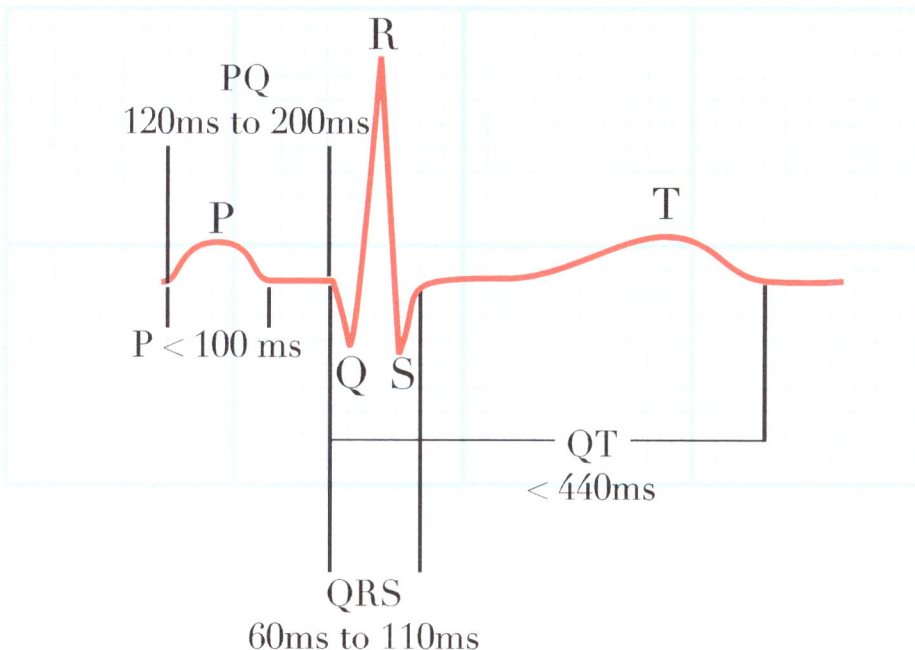

Figure 17: Electrocardiographic intervals.

Chronology is an important element in the ECG diagnosis. The A-V conduction time is first determined and is measured from the beginning of the P wave to the first deflection of the QRS complex; it is the PQ (or PR) interval. It depends essentially on the conduction velocity through the A-V node but in fact includes the conduction through the atrium and the His-Purkinje fibers. It is usually 120 to 200 ms long. Q wave duration should be < 40 ms (except in III and aVR) its amplitude < 25% of the QRS complex (excepted in III and aVR). QRS duration is between 60 ms and 110 ms. Repolarisation duration is calculated between the beginning of the QRS complex and the end of the T wave. The QT interval needs some correction because it varies with heart rate. Its value is between 320 ms and 440 ms (Figs. **17** and **19**). Micropotentials of the QRS complex are defined when its amplitude is < 5 mm in the limb leads and < 10 mm in the precordial leads. By convention, cardiac activation chronology can be represented as follows (Fig. **18**): 1) represents the sino-atrial conduction (not visible on the surface ECG), 2) represents the atrial activation, 3) represents the A-V conduction and 4) represents the ventricular activation.

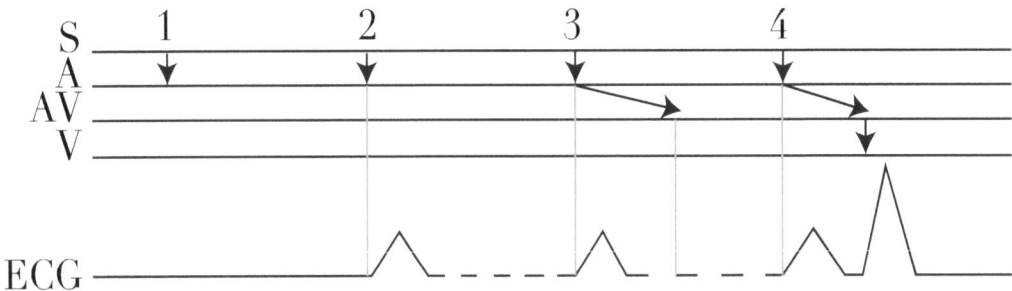

Figure 18: Chronology of cardiac activation.

THE ELECTRICAL AXIS

Frontal Electrical Axis

The electrical axis refers to the general direction of the heart's depolarisation wavefront (or mean electrical vector) in the frontal plane. It is the algebraic sum of the various QRS components in the front plan (Fig. **20**). It is perpendicular to the derivation where this sum equals zero, which is rare. The following example shows how to calculate the axis. Example: if the algebraic sum is zero in aVL and maximal in II, this axis is +60° [6].

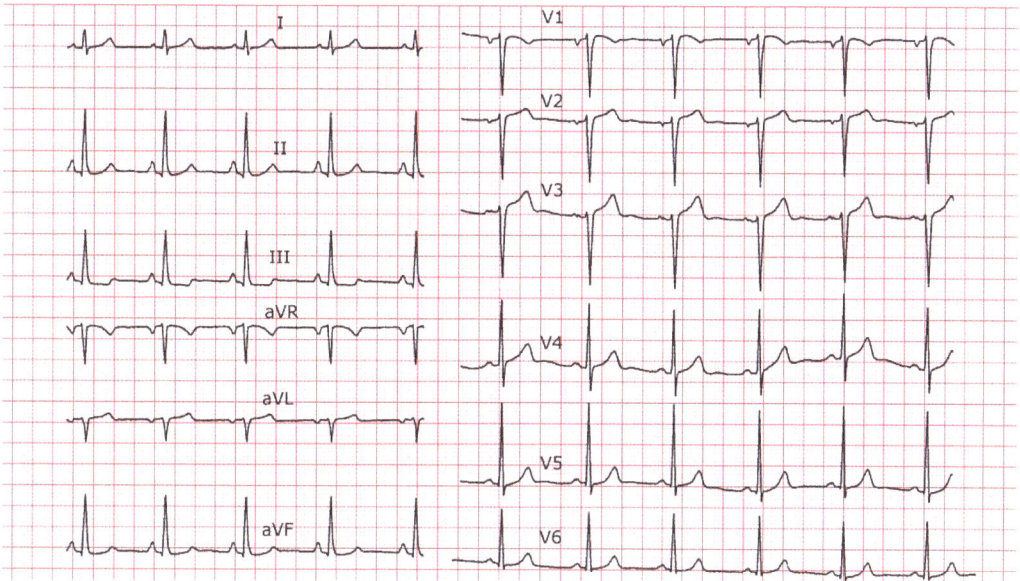

Figure 19: Normal ECG trace.

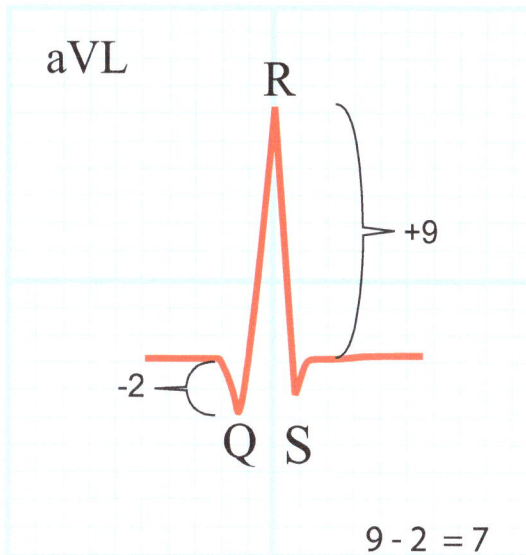

Figure 20: Electrical axis determination.

If the sum equal zero in aVF, the axis is parallel to the derivation perpendicular to aVF, I. If the sum is sligthly positive in aVF, the axis will be more vertical somewhere between 0 and +30°. In clinical practice the axis is mainly determined by using the polarity in the 2 leads, I and aVF; then the isoelectric lead is used to more precisely calculate the axis. Axis determination, in the presence of conduction abnormalities, (especially right bundle branch block), should be done by using only the first 60 ms of the QRS complex.

Horizontal Electrical Axis

As mentionned previously, the electrical transition in the horizontal plane occurs in the precordial leads between V3 and V4 and corresponds to the interventricular septal position. Counterclockwise rotation means that the rotation occurs in V1 or V2 and is due to a left deviation of the interventricular septum. Late transition or clockwise transition occurs in V5 or V6.

Heart Rate

In principle, the paper speed of the electrocardiogramm is 25 mm per second. Knowing that each division equals 1 mm or 40 ms, heart rate can easily be calculated. If 14 small squares separate 2 QRS (or P waves), the RR or PP interval is: 14 x 40 = 560 ms. Heart rate is obtained by dividing the number of ms in 1 minute by the calculated interval: 60000 / 560 = 107 beats per minute (bpm). With great variation of the heart rate the mean heart rate is calculated with an average of 6 to 8 RR intervals (Fig. **21**) [12].

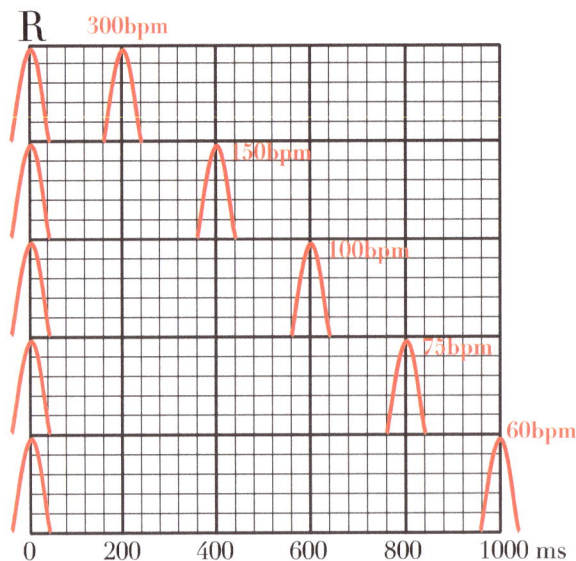

Figure 21: Heart rate calculation.

THE NORMAL SINUS RHYTHM

In sinus rhythm, depolarisation is transmitted to the atrium and afterwards to the ventricle. On the surface ECG the consequences are a positive P wave in all derivations except aVR, a constant PR interval and a regular RR interval equal to the PP interval. At rest, the heart rate is around 60 bpm with a slight variation due to respiratory activity. A heart rate < 60 bpm is called bradycardia and a heart rate > 100 bpm is called tachycardia. With high heart rate the P waves are sometimes non visible because they are concealed in the preceding T wave [1,3].

ACKNOWLEDGEMENT

Declared none.

CONFLICT OF INTEREST

The author(s) confirm that this chapter content has no conflict of interest.

REFERENCES

[1]   Mirvis DM: Physiology and biophysics in electrocardiography. J Electrocardiol 29:175-177, 1996.
[2]   Braunwald's Heart Disease : A Textbook of Cardiovascular Medicine: Elsevier- Saunders, 2011.
[3]   Fye WB: A history of the origin, evolution, and impact of electrocardiography. Am J Cardiol 73:937-949, 1994.
[4]   Fisch C: Centennial of the string galvanometer and the electrocardiogram. J Am Coll Cardiol 26:1737-1742, 2000.
[5]   Barr RC: Genesis of the electrocardiogram. In MacFarlane PW, Lawrie TDV (eds): Comprehensive Electrocardiography: Theory and Practice in Health and Disease. New York, Pergamon, 1989.
[6]   Zywitz C: Technical aspects of the electrocardiographic recording. In MacFarlane PW, Lawrie TDV (eds): Comprehensive Electrocardiography. New York, Pergamon, 1989.
[7]   Bailey JJ, Berson AS, Garson A, *et al.* Recommendations and specifications in automated electrocardiography: Bandwidth and digital signal processing. Circulation 81:730-739, 1990.
[8]   Debbas NMG, Jackson SHD, de Jonghe D, *et al.* Human atrial depolarization: Effects of sinus rate, pacing and drugs on the surface electrocardiogram. J Am Coll Cardiol 33:358-365, 1999.
[9]   Janse MJ: Propagation of atrial impulses through the atrioventricular node. In Toubol P, Waldo AL (eds): Atrial Arrhythmias. St Louis, Mosby-Year Book, 1990.

[10]   Franz MR, Bargheer K, Costartd-Jackle A, *et al.* Human ventricular repolarization and T wave genesis. Prog Cardiovasc Dis 33:369-384, 1991.

[11]   Durrer D, van Dam RT, Freud GF, *et al.* Total excitation of the human heart. Circulation 41:899-912, 1970.

[12]   Vitelli LL, Crow RS, Shahar E, *et al.* Electrocardiographic findings in a healthy biracial population. Am J Cardiol 81:453-459, 1998.

Send Orders of Reprints at reprints@benthamscience.net
Electrocardiography (ECG), 2013, 23-26

CHAPTER 2

ECG Analysis

Abstract: A systematic analysis of the surface ECG is crucial in the diagnostic process (Fig. **1**). A good description allows comprehension of the trace and definition of the problem [1-4]. Paper speed and dimensions of grids on ECG paper have to be checked. The rhythm should be precisely defined. If it is not sinus rhythm the following criteria are useful to aid rhythm determination. The heart rate is usually calculated during determination of the rhythm. A small square represents 40 ms. When heart rate is below 60 bpm it is a bradycardia and when it is over 100 bpm it is a tachycardia. The duration, the axis and the morphology of the P wave have to be carefully checked. The P-R interval is the time required for completion of atrial depolarisation; conduction through the A-V node, His bundle and bundle branches; and arrival at the ventricular myocardial cells. Its value is between 120 and 200 ms. The duration, the axis, the morphology and the presence of Q waves should be evaluated. Abnormal Q waves have a duration > 40 ms and an amplitude of at least 25% of the QRS complex. Position of the ST segment should be checked to detect elevation or depression. Non specific changes should be placed in the clinical context. The T wave can be positive, negative or flat. It must also be analyzed within the clinical context. Conduction abnormalities will also modify the T wave and we should not forget that when depolarisation is abnormal, repolarisation is also abnormal. It is measured from the beginning of the QRS complex to the end of the T wave. QT interval duration varies with heart rate and shortens with tachycardia. Its correct value can be calculated with the Bazett formula.

Keywords: Cardiac rhythm, heart rate, sinus rhythm, P wave, T wave, QRS complex, PQ interval, QRS interval, QRS complex duration, QRS complex amplitude.

PAPER SPEED AND DIMENSIONS OF GRIDS ON ECG PAPER

The paper speed is 25 mm/s. Amplitude of the waves is represented by blocks 1mV=10 small squares.

RHYTHM [5]

The rhythm should be precisely defined. If it is not sinus rhythm the following criteria are useful to aid rhythm determination.

Two criteria define sinus rhythm:

1. Presence of P waves.

2. Positive P waves in leads I, and II (between 0 and 75°), negative in aVR.

Jean-Jacques Goy, Jean-Christophe Stauffer, Jürg Schlaepfer and Pierre Christeler

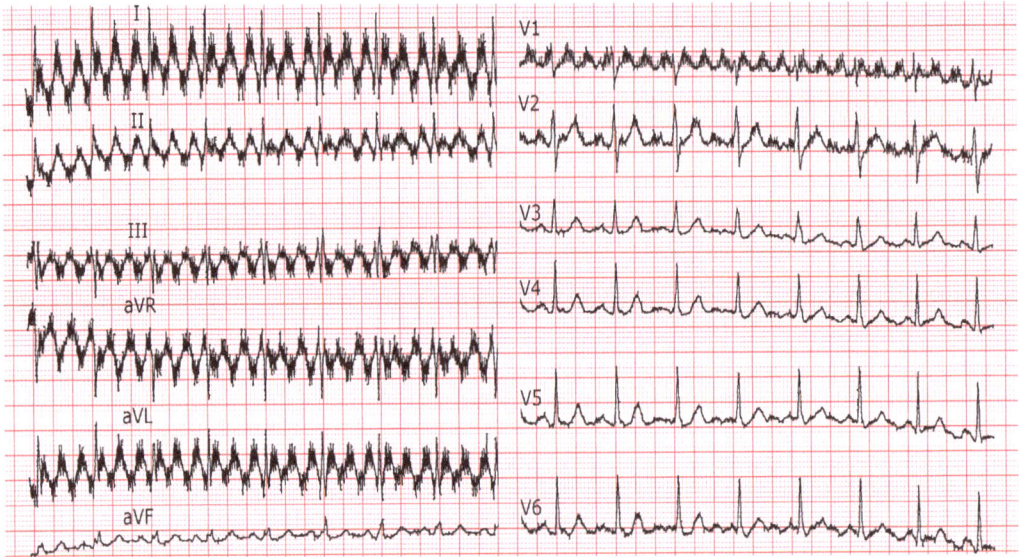

Figure 1: Electrical artifact. The diagnosis is evident provided a careful and rigorous analysis is done.

If the rhythm is not sinus rhythm, the position and the axis of the P waves help in the diagnosis. The P waves can be:

1. Absent because of sinus arrest.

2. Absent and replaced by atrial flutter or fibrillation waves.

3. Absent because they are hidden in the QRS complex.

4. Present between the QRS complexes. In a narrow QRS tachycardia the relationship between P' waves and QRS omplexes is useful to determine the mechanism of the tachycardia.

5. Present but completely dissociated from the QRS complexes (A-V dissociation) as seen in complete A-V block or ventricular tachycardia.

RATE ANALYSIS [5]

The heart rate is usually calculated during determination of the rhythm. A small square represents 40 ms. When heart rate is below 60 bpm it is a bradycardia and when it is over 100 bpm it is a tachycardia.

P WAVE ANALYSIS [5]

The duration, the axis and the morphology of the P wave have to be carefully checked.

PR OR PQ INTERVAL [5]

The P-R interval is the time required for completion of atrial depolarisation; conduction through the A-V node, His bundle and bundle branches; and arrival at the ventricular myocardial cells. Its value is between 120 and 200 m.

QRS ANALYSIS [5]

The duration, the axis, the morphology and the presence of Q waves should be evaluated. Abnormal Q waves have duration > 40 ms and amplitude of at least 25% of the QRS complex.

ST SEGMENT ANALYSIS [5]

Its position should be checked to detect elevation or depression. Non specific changes should be placed in the clinical context.

T WAVE [5]

The T wave can be positive, negative or flat. It must also be analyzed within the clinical context. Conduction abnormalities will also modify the T wave and we should not forget that when depolarisation is abnormal, repolarisation is also abnormal.

QT INTERVAL [5]

It is measured from the beginning of the QRS complex to the end of the T wave. Its duration varies with heart rate and shortens with tachycardia. Its correct value can be calculated with the Bazett formula.

Normal Values

P wave	Maximal duration: <100 ms, axis: 0-75° Amplitude: < 2.5 mm in II and III PQ interval: ≥ 120 ms and ≤ 200 ms
PQ interval	≥ 120 ms and ≤ 200 ms
QRS complex	Maximal duration: ≤110 ms, axis: between -30° and +90° pathological Q waves: 25% more of the QRS amplitude
QT interval	QTC < 440 ms

ACKNOWLEDGEMENT

Declared none.

CONFLICT OF INTEREST

The author(s) confirm that this chapter content has no conflict of interest.

REFERENCES

[1]   Chou T-C, Knilans TK: Electrocardiography in Clinical Practice: Adult and Pediatric. 4th ed. Philadelphia, WB Saunders, 1996.

[2]   Schlant RC, Adolph RJ, DiMarco JP, *et al.* Guidelines for electrocardiography. A report of the American College of Cardiology/American Heart Association Task Force on Assessment of Diagnostic and Therapeutic Cardiovascular Procedures (Committee on Electrocardiography). Circulation 85:1221-1228, 1992

[3]   MacFarlane PW, Lawrie TDV (eds): Comprehensive Electrocardiology: Theory and Practice in Health and Disease. Vol 3. New York, Pergamon, 1989.

[4]   Franz MR: Time for yet another QT correction algorithm? Bazett and beyond. J Am Coll Cardiol 23:1554-1557, 1994.

[5]   Kennedy HL, Goldberger AL, Graboys TB, *et al.* American College of Cardiology guidelines for training in adult cardiovascular medicine. Task Force 2: Training in electrocardiography, ambulatory electrocardiography, and exercise testing. J Am Coll Cardiol 25:1013, 1995.

CHAPTER 3

Conduction Abnormalities

Abstract: In this chapter, we address the basic notions of conduction abnormalities. Impairment can occur in any part of the conduction system. Prolongation of the PR interval over 200 ms is the characteristic feature of first degree A-V block. Second degree A-V block includes Wenckebach, Mobitz II A-V block and 2:1 A-V block. The characteristic ECG feature of Wenckebach block, also called Mobitz I, is progressive lengthening of the PR interval until finally a beat is dropped. This is a more severe form of second degree block. The characteristic ECG picture is that of a series of one or more non-conducted P waves, 2:1, 3:1, 4:1 block. Two to one A-V block (2:1 block) can be of the types Mobitz I or II. It can be nodal or infra-hisian. A P wave is conducted, the following one is blocked and so on. Third degree A-V block, also known as complete A-V block, is a complete disruption of A-V conduction. The atria and the ventricles are paced independently. Block of conduction in the left bundle branch, prior to its bifurcation, results primarily in delayed depolarisation of the left ventricle. In LBBB, the septum depolarizes from right to left, since in this case depolarisation is initiated by the right bundle branch. In rigth bundle branch block (RBBB) conduction along the right branch of the His bundle no longer exists. The ventricles are activated only by the left branch.

Sinus activity is not visible on the surface ECG. Thus first degree sino-atrial block is only theoretical without electrophysiological sequelae. Only second and third degree sino-atrial blocks are visible on the surface ECG and these do have some clinical importance. Second degree block of the type Wenckebach occurs with a progressive shortening of the PP interval and a slight increase of the heart rate followed by a pause with a duration greater than the PP interval preceding it but less than the next PP interval. Third degree block or complete block cannot be distinguished at all from true atrial standstill: absence of atrial activity, His bundle escape rhythm with narrow QRS complexes and sometimes retrograde P' waves with a polarity opposite to sinus P wave polarity. The pacemaker rhythm can easily be recognized on the ECG. It shows pacemaker spikes: vertical artifact signals that represent the electrical activity of the pacemaker. Usually these spikes are more visible in unipolar than in bipolar pacing. The morphology of the QRS complex helps to locate the site of ventricular pacing, typically right bundle branch block morphology for left ventricular pacing and left bundle branch block morphology for right ventricular pacing.

Keywords: Sino-atrial block, atrio-ventricular block, left bundle branch block, rigth bundle branch block, left anterior hemiblock, left posterior hemiblock, second degree atrioventricular block, first degree atrio-ventricular block, Mobitz I block, Mobitz II block, complete atrio-ventricular block.

Jean-Jacques Goy, Jean-Christophe Stauffer, Jürg Schlaepfer and Pierre Christeler

A-V CONDUCTION ABNORMALITIES (ATRIO-VENTRICULAR)

Impairment can occur in any part of the conduction system. We should remember that the true A-V conduction system represents depolarisation through the A-V node and the His bundle only. However, on the surface ECG, A-V conduction includes atrial activation [1-5].

The etiology of conduction abnormalities is multiple: from conduction pathway sclerosis, cardiomyopathy, ischemic heart disease, electrolytic disturbances, to drug toxicity like digitalis.

There are 3 types of block, classified by grade of block (Fig. **1**):

1.   At suprahisian level including the A-V node.

2.   At intrahisian level within the trunk of the His bundle.

3.   At infrahisian level concurrently within the right and the left bundle branches.

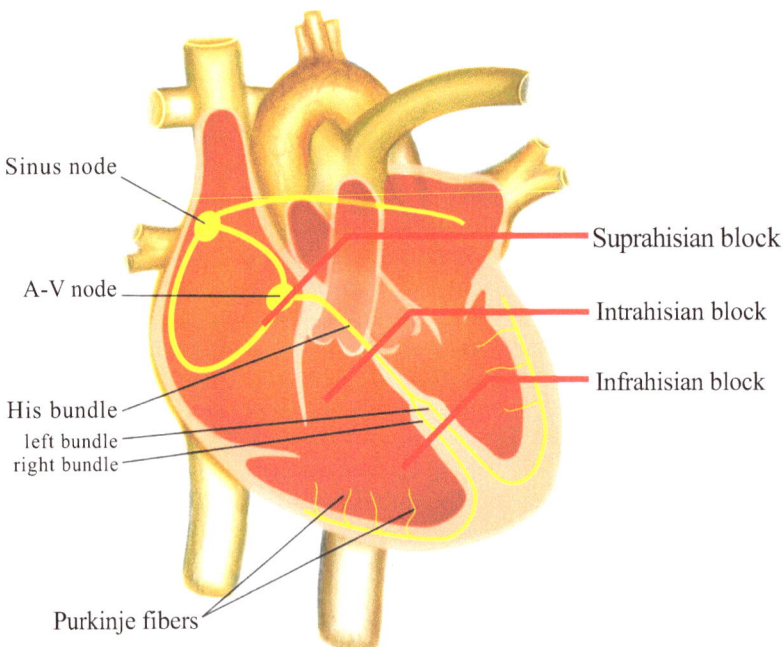

Figure 1: Location of the A-V block.

First Degree A-V Block

Prolongation of the PR interval over 200 ms is the characteristic feature of first degree A-V block. It is, in fact, not a true block but only a delayed conduction. Practically, the PR interval is measured from the beginning of the P wave to the first deflection of the QRS complex (Q or R wave). It includes the conduction time through the atrium, the A-V node and the His bundle. In some leads, the initial portion of the P wave can be isoelectric making the PR interval erroneously short. Thus the PR interval has to be measured in the lead where it is the longest (Figs. **2** and **3**). This block is usually located within the A-V node [1-6].

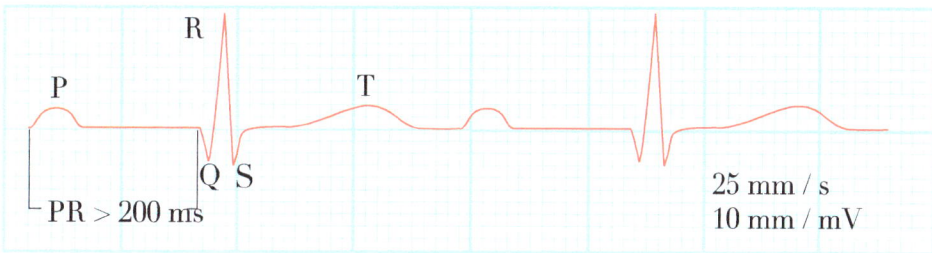

Figure 2: First degree A-V block.

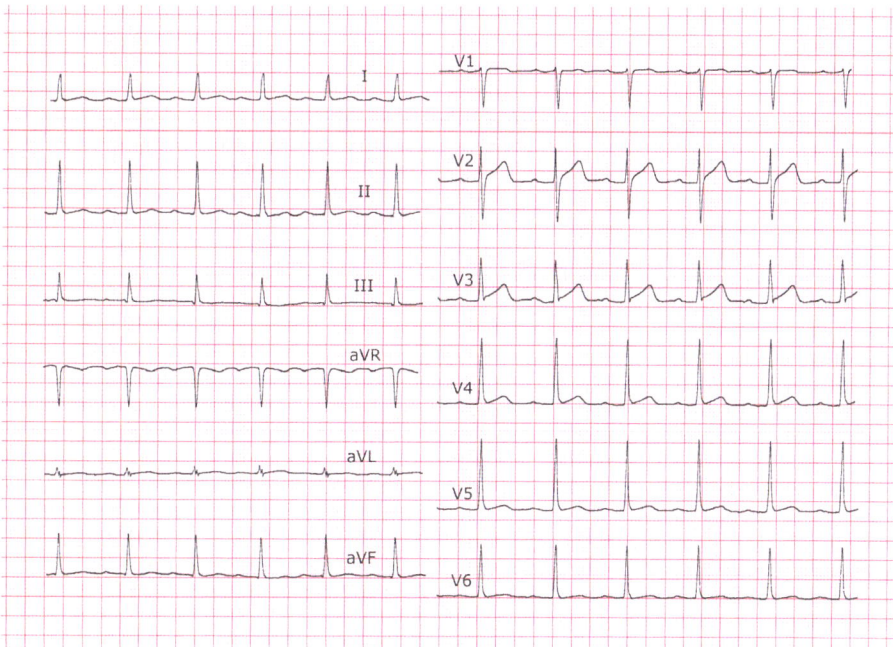

Figure 3: Sinus rhythm with a prolonged PQ interval (240 ms) typical of first degree A-V block.

Second Degree A-V Block

There are 2 types (Fig. **4**).

Second Degree A-V Block Type Wenckebach or Mobitz I

The characteristic ECG feature of Wenckebach block, also called Mobitz I, is progressive lengthening of the PR interval until finally a beat is dropped. The dropped beat is seen as a P wave that is not followed by a QRS complex. The phenomenon repeats itself in longer or shorter sequences. This block is usually seen when the heart rate is increased (Figs. **4** and **5**). The Wenckebach phenomenon has 4 characteristics: 1) a first normal or slightly prolonged PR interval. 2) a progressive lengthening (over 3 or 4 cycles) of the PR interval 3) finally a blocked P wave 4) a shortening of the RR intervals preceding the blocked P wave with a slightly increased heart rate [1-5].

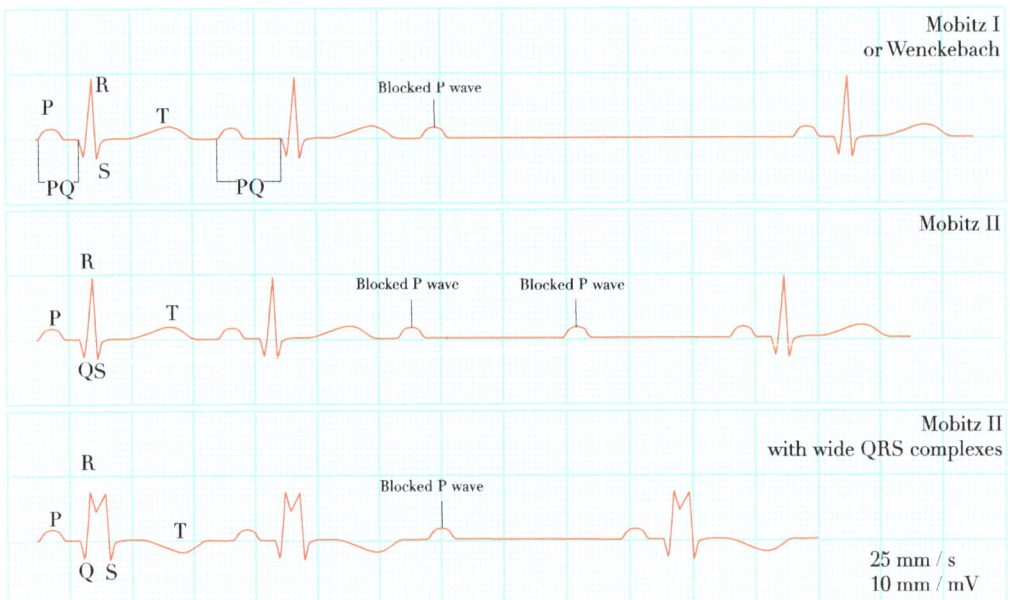

Figure 4: Second degree A-V block.

Second Degree A-V Block Type Mobitz II

This is a more severe form of second degree block. The characteristic ECG picture is that of a series of one or more non-conducted P waves, 2:1, 3:1, 4:1

block. The atrial activity remains regular and also ventriculo-phasic arrhythmia can be seen. This means that P-P intervals flanking a QRS complex are shorter than those which do not. Quite often, there is associated bundle branch block and the QRS complex is wide. The cause is usually an infra-hisian block (Figs. **6** and **7**) [1-6].

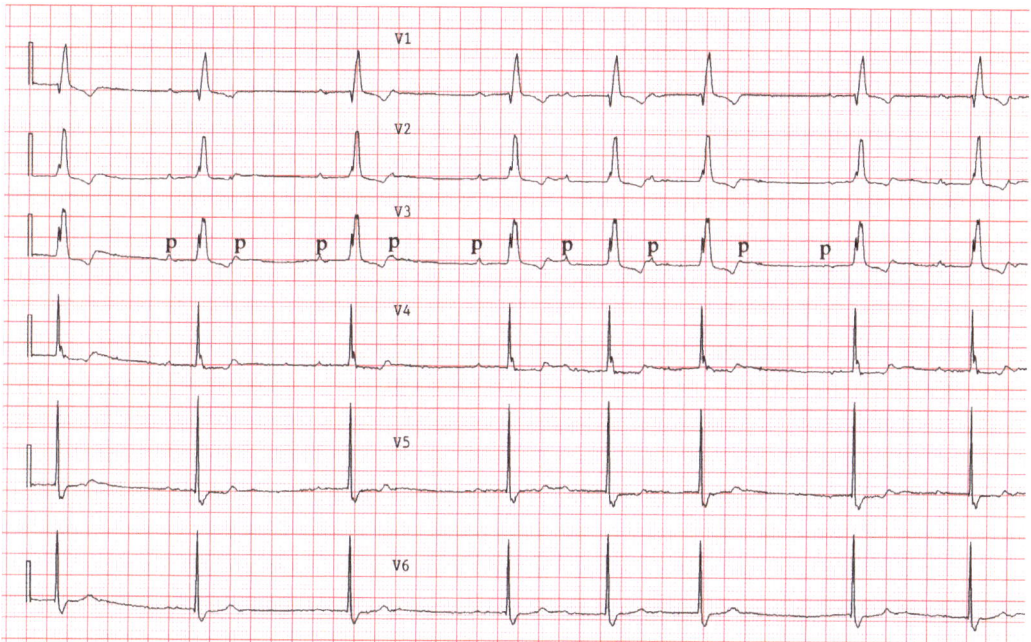

Figure 5: Sinus rhythm with 2:1 A-V block on the left side of the trace and with second degree A-V block type Wenckebach on the right side.

Special Case of the 2:1 A-V Block

Two to one A-V block (2:1 block) can be of the types Mobitz I or II. It can be nodal or infra-hisian. A P wave is conducted, the following one is blocked and so on. The number of blocked P waves is the same as the number of conducted P waves. There are twice as many P waves as QRS complexes (Fig. **6**) [2, 4, 5].

Third Degree A-V Block or Complete A-V Block [1-3]

Third degree A-V block, also known as complete A-V block, is a complete disruption of A-V conduction. The atria and the ventricles are paced independently. P waves are present and occur at a rate faster than the ventricular rate; QRS complexes are present and occur at a regular rate, usually 40 to 50 bpm; the P waves bear no relationship to the QRS complexes [2, 4, 5].

In other words, 2 separate rhythms coexist: on the one hand atrial activity (P waves) and on the other hand ventricular activity (QRS complexes) (Figs. **7, 8** and **9**). At the start of the episode of complete A-V block, ventricular escape may not be immediate, leading to clinical symptoms such as syncope.

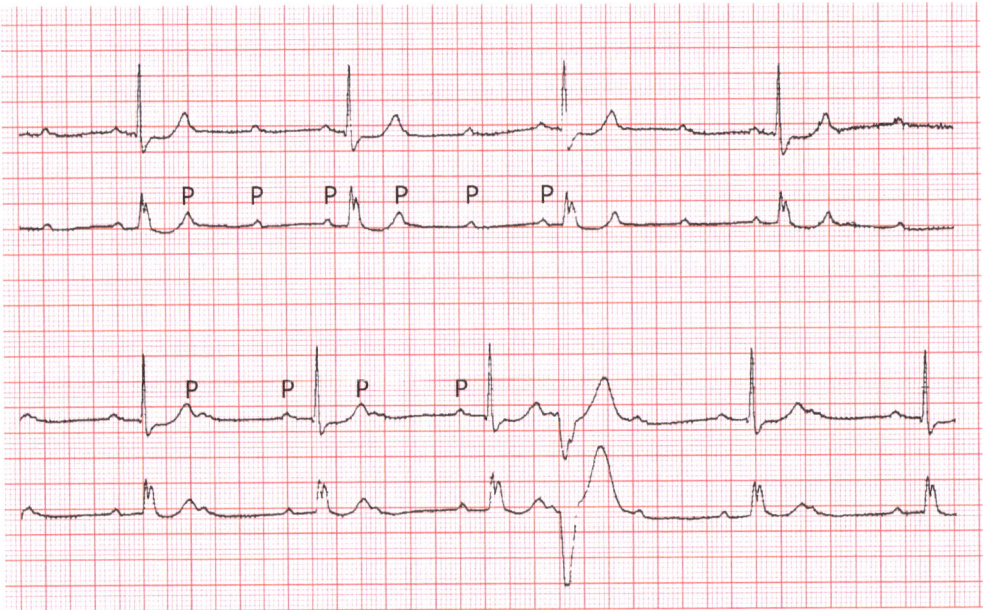

Figure 6: Second degree A-V block type Mobitz II. In the upper trace one P wave in 3 is conducted to the ventricles (conduction 3:1). In the lower trace one P wave in 2 is conducted (conduction 2:1 = A-V block 2:1). The ventricular premature beat is coincidental.

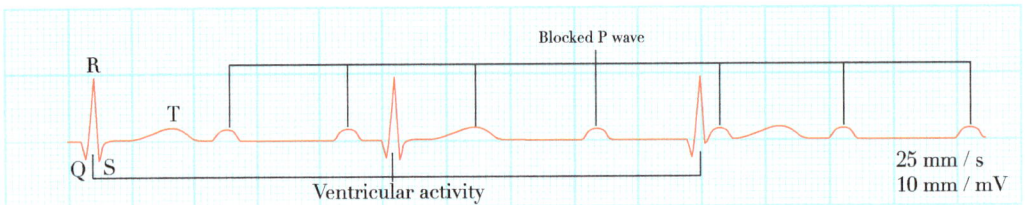

Figure 7: Complete A-V block with dissociation between the P waves and the QRS complexes

Complete A-V block can be present even if the baseline rhythm is not sinus rhythm. This can be observed with atrial fibrillation or atrial flutter. In this case they are no P waves but only oscillations of the baseline, typical of atrial fibrillation, but with regular QRS complexes (Fig. **10**).

Anatomical Location of the Block

The location of the block may have therapeutic implications. The electrocardiographic appearance depends on the site of the block and on the escape rhythm.

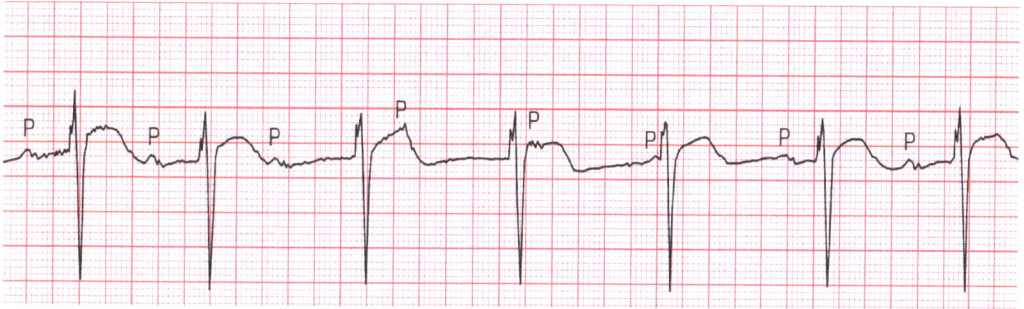

Figure 8: Complete A-V block with dissociation between the P waves and the (wide) QRS complexes.

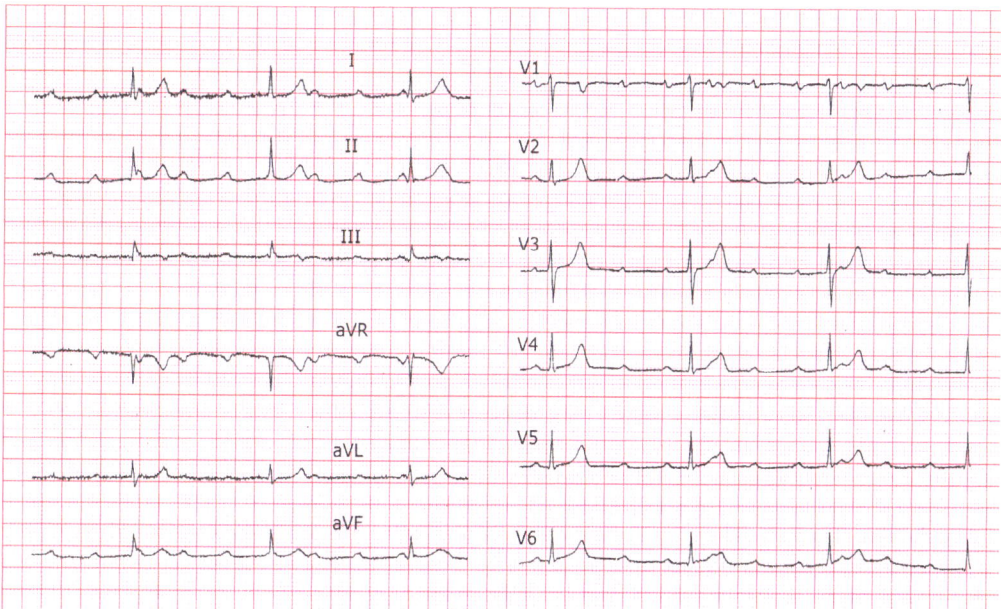

Figure 9: Sinus rhythm with dissociation between the P waves and the QRS complexes. The QRS complexes from the escape rhythm are narrow. Therefore this escape rhythm arises from the A-V node.

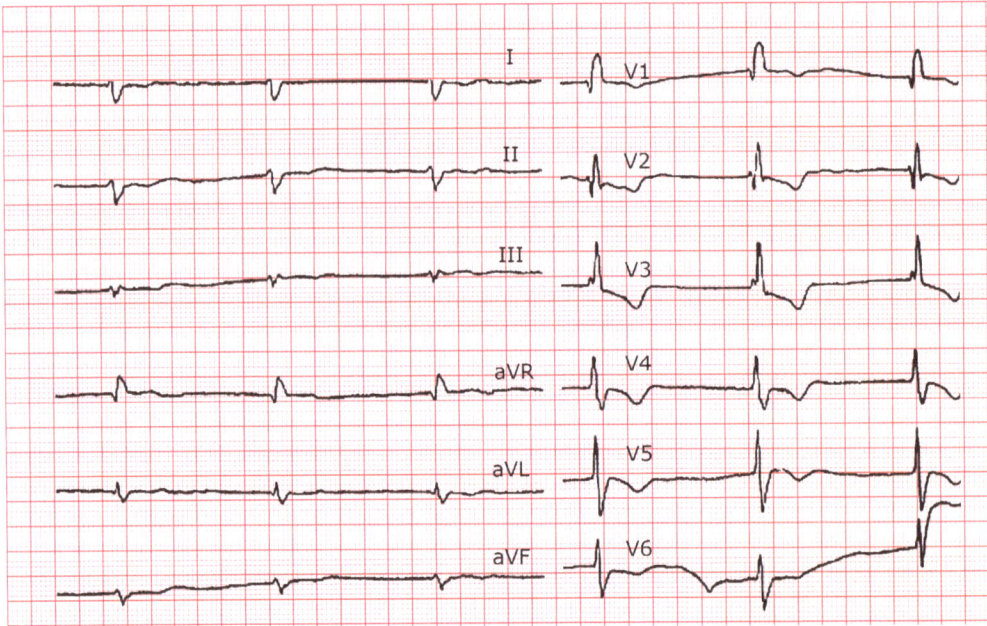

Figure 10: The baseline rhythm is atrial fibrillation (AF). The QRS complexes are regular because of complete A-V block. The QRS complexes are large because of the presence of right bundle branch block.

Suprahisian Block

The escape rhythm arises from the A-V node or the His bundle. In these 2 situations, the depolarisation goes through the His bundle trunk and then simultaneously through the 2 branches as with normal A-V conduction. The QRS complexes are narrow unless a preexisting bundle branch block is present and prolongs its duration (Fig. **11**).

Intrahisian Block

The escape rhythm arises from the distal part of the trunk of the left bundle with a simultaneous depolarisation of the branches as for suprahisian block. The QRS complex remains narrow unless a preexisting bundle branch block is present.

Infrahissian Block

A simultaneous block of the 2 branches of the His bundle results in an infrahisian block. The escape rhythm, always localized below the lesion, arises from the distal portion of one of the branches or even below, in the ventricles. If the source of the escape rhythm is located in a hemibranch, the QRS complex exhibits the same pattern as contralateral hemiblock. For example, an escape rhythm arising from the left anterior hemibranch will produce a QRS complex morphology of RBBB and left posterior hemiblock. If it is located more distally in the ventricle, the escape rhythm will have a wide QRS complex completely different from a LBBB or RBBB. This rhythm is called "idioventricular" (Fig. **12**).

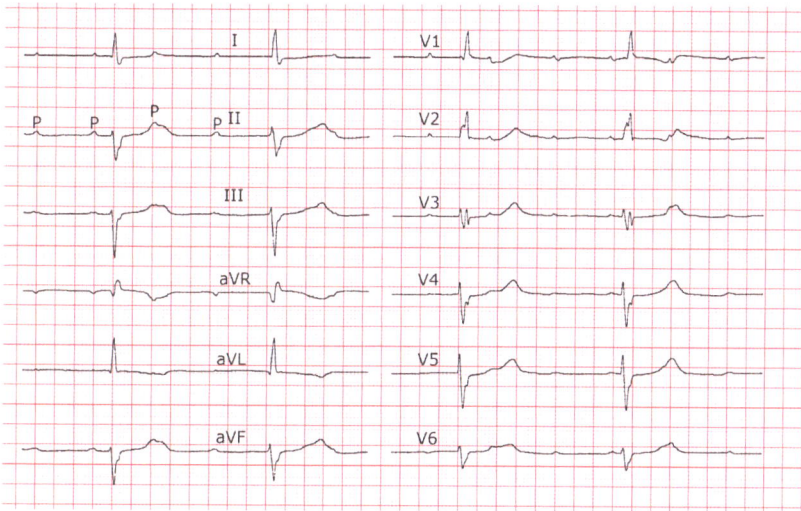

Figure 11: Sinus rhythm with complete dissociation between the P waves and the QRS complexes. The escape rhythm is either, nodal with RBBB and left anterior hemiblock or arises from the posterior branch of the left bundle.

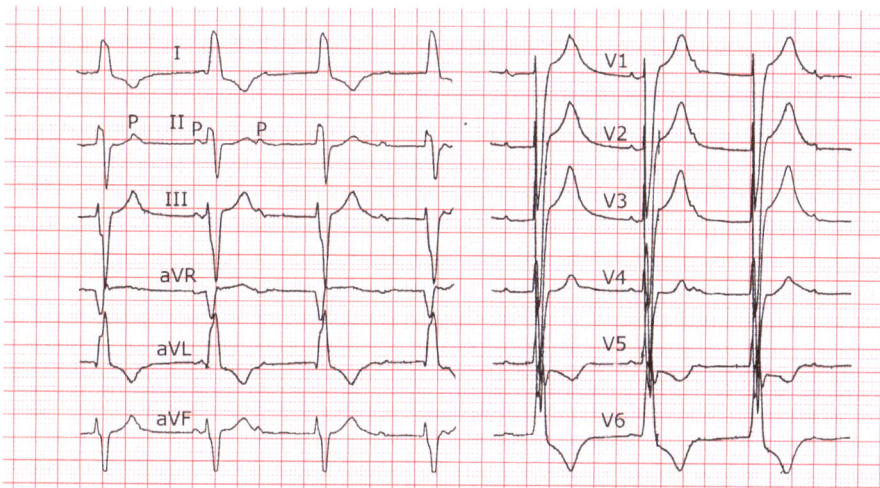

Figure 12: Complete A-V block with ventricular escape rhythm.

Diagnostic Criteria

Distinction between suprahisian and intrahisian block is impossible on the surface ECG. However A-V block with narrow QRS complex is more often intrahisian than suprahisian (nodal). Wide QRS complex without the appearance of LBBB or RBBB is almost always infrahisian. Very often, it is only possible to determine the precise localization of block with endocardial electrograms.

Narrow QRS Complex

The block is usually suprahisian, nodal or intrahisian.

Wide QRS Complexes with LBBB Morphology

It is usually an infrahisian block. A preexisting unilateral bundle branch block with a secondary bundle branch block results in complete A-V block. In some cases, nodal or intrahisian block can be associated with a wide QRS complex if proximal A-V block coexists with bundle branch block. Finally, when the QRS complex is very prolonged with a morphology incompatible with a classical bundle branch block, the escape rhythm is located in the ventricle and the rhythm is called idioventricular.

INTRAVENTRICULAR CONDUCTION DISTURBANCES

In the normal process of ventricular depolarisation, the electrical stimulus reaches the ventricles *via* the atrioventricular (A-V) junction. Then the depolarisation wave spreads to the main mass of the ventricular muscle *via* the right and left bundle branches. Normally the entire process of ventricular depolarisation occurs in less than 100 ms. Any process that interferes with the normal depolarisation of the ventricles may prolong the QRS width because the depolarisation propagates through the ventricular muscles and take more time to depolarize the 2 ventricles. Usually the QRS duration is ≥ 120 ms [6-8].

Left Bundle Branch Block (LBBB)

Block of conduction in the left bundle branch, prior to its bifurcation, results primarily in delayed depolarisation of the left ventricle. In LBBB, the septum depolarizes from right to left, since in this case depolarisation is initiated by the right bundle branch. Next, the right ventricle depolarizes, followed by delayed depolarisation of the left ventricle, giving an R-R1 configuration in lead V6 and a QRS interval of greater than 0.12 seconds. Hence, LBBB is characterized by an R-R1 configuration in lead V6 and a QRS interval > 120 ms. A q wave in V6 (and in I) represents normal septal activation. As the septal activation is reversed this q wave is not present with LBBB. Because of the abnormally slow progression of the depolarisation, the activation of the left ventricle is delayed compared to right ventricular depolarisation. This causes a "ventricular dyssynchrony" (which is visible on the ECG.) with an initial positivity in V6 without a q wave. In V1 a wide and deep S wave sometimes preceded by a small r wave; otherwise the QRS is a QS complex). Then the activation goes from the right to the left part of the septum causing a delayed depolarisation and therefore a prolongation of the QRS duration >120 ms. The QRS is deeply negative in V1 and exclusively positive in V6). The left free wall activation is normal and the left ventricular activation ends with a final positive wave in V6). Repolarisation is in the opposite direction to depolarisation and visible as a negative T wave in the left precordial leads (Figs. **13** and **14**) [6, 7, 9].

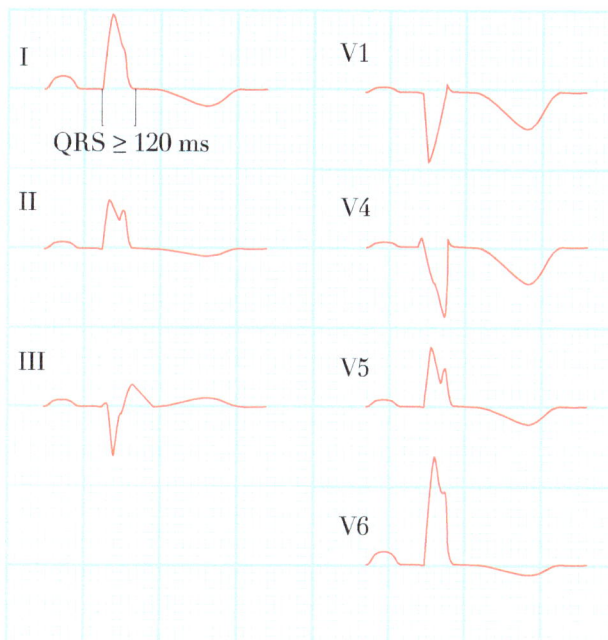

Figure 13: Complete left bundle branch block.

Left bundle branch block criteria (LBBB) [3, 11]:

- QRS duration ≥ 120 ms.

- Deformation of the QRS complex due to ventricular dyssynchrony: wide R wave in V6, rS or QS appearance in V1.

- Wide QRS complex with duration proportional to the degree of block.

- T wave inversion in V5 and V6.

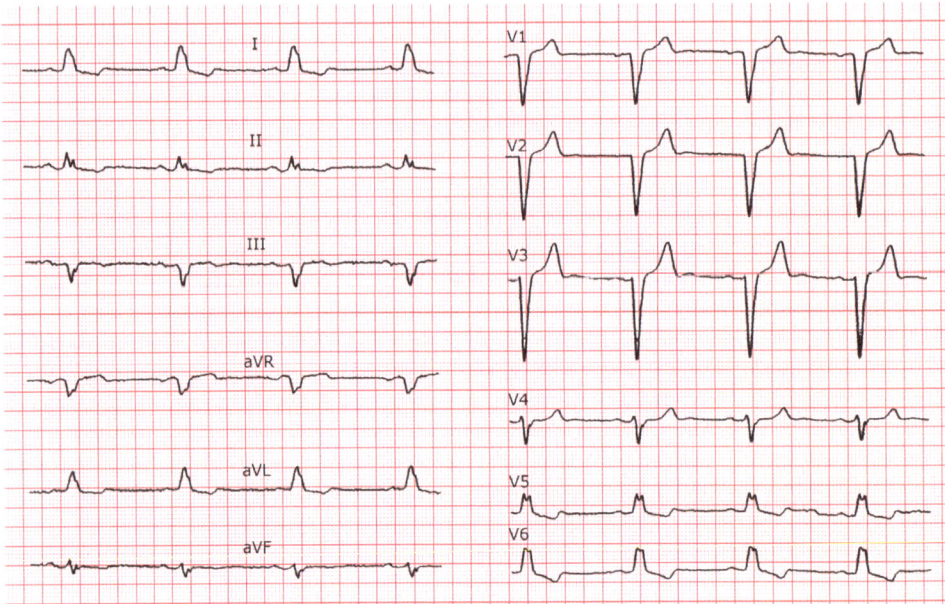

Figure 14: Typical appearance of left bundle branch block.

Incomplete left bundle branch block occurs when depolarisation is not blocked but only slowed. The QRS complex exhibits the modifications of the LBBB but less marked and with a duration of 110 ms. Its morphology is between the normal QRS complex and the QRS morphology of the LBBB.

Left Anterior Hemiblock

Conduction block occurs in the anterior branches (fascicles) of the left bundle branch. The main effect of a fascicular block is to markedly change the QRS axis

(> - 30°) without changing the shape or duration of the QRS wave form. A small q wave is present in I, a deep S wave in the limb leads (II, III, aVF), and a mirror image of a tall R wave in the lateral leads (I and aVL), in the precordial leads, the zone of transition is displaced laterally with a deep S wave in V6 (Fig. **15**) [5].

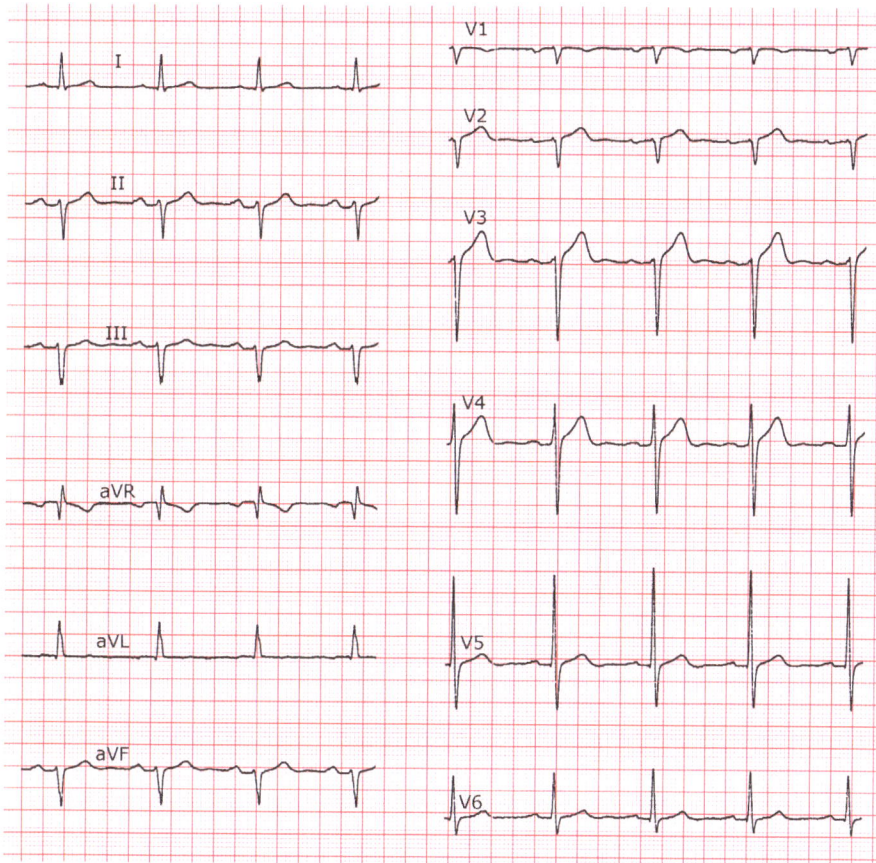

Figure 15: Left anterior hemiblock, with left axis deviation and deep S waves in II, III and aVF.

Criteria of left anterior hemiblock [3, 5, 10, 11]:

-   Normal QRS morphology in the precordial leads with an s wave in V6.

-   qR appearance in I, rS in II and III (deep S waves).

-   Left axis deviation in the frontal plane (> -30°).

- S wave in V 6.

Left Posterior Hemiblock

Here, conduction block occurs in the posterior branches (fascicles) of the left bundle branch. This results in right axis deviation ($\geq 90°$). A deep S wave is present in I and aVL, with tall R waves in II, III and aVF preceded by a small q wave in the inferior leads (S1, q3) (Fig. **16**) [3, 5, 10].

Criteria of left posterior hemiblock [3, 5, 6]:

- rS appearance in I and aVL

- qR in II and III (Tall T waves).

- Right axis deviation.

- Normal precordial leads.

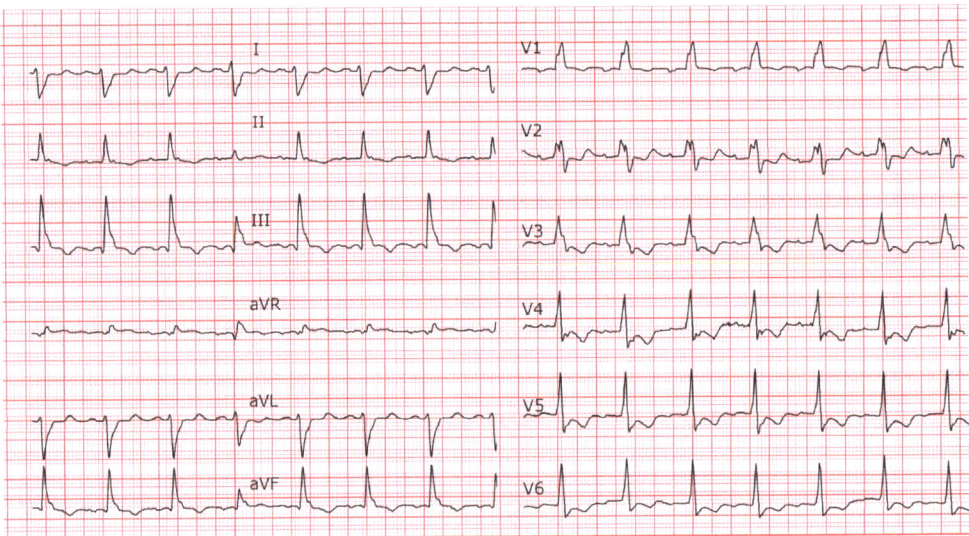

Figure 16: Left posterior hemiblock and RBBB.

Complete Right Bundle Branch Block (RBBB)

Conduction along the right branch of the His bundle no longer exists. The ventricles are activated only by the left branch: 1) the beginning of the ventricular activation is unchanged: septal depolarisation results in a small R wave in V, corresponding to the small negative initial depolarisation in V6 (q wave). The vectors of the left ventricular activation are unchanged in V6 with a positive R wave, and a negative S wave in V1. 2) There after the activation goes from left to right to reach the right branch of the His bundle. 3) then the right side of the septum and the free wall of the right ventricle are activated. This gives a positive deflection in V1 (R' wave) and a negative deflection in V6 (S wave) slightly broadened in I and V6 (Figs. **17** and **18**) [5, 9].

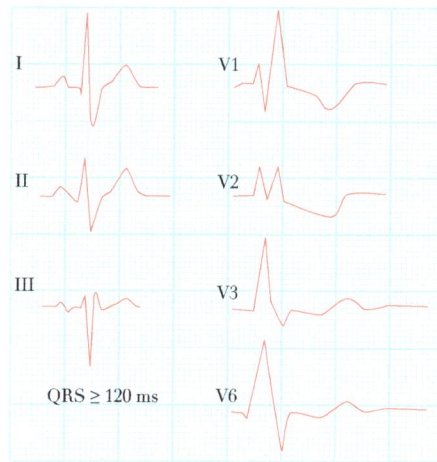

Figure 17: Complete right bundle branch block.

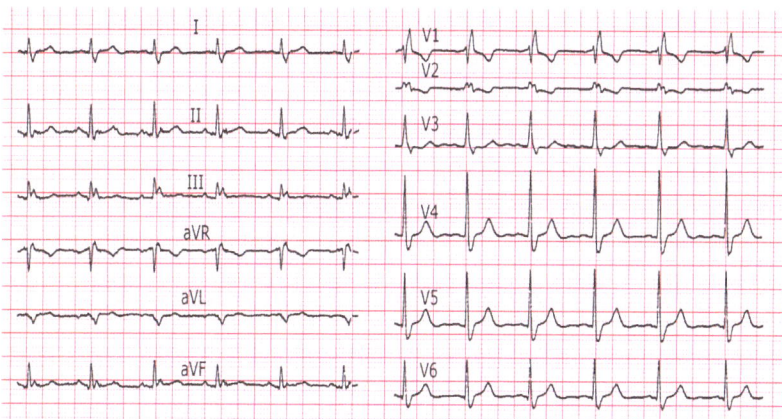

Figure 18: Sinus rhythm with complete right bundle branch block (rsR' in V1, QRS > 120 ms, deep S waves in V6).

Criteria of complete right bundle branch block (RBBB):

- QRS duration ≥ 120 ms.

- Unmodified ventricular activation (persistent r wave in V1 and q wave in V6).

- Modification of the terminal portion of the ventricular activation with a second positivity in V1 and a terminal negativity in V6 due to the delayed depolarisation of the right ventricle.

- QRS morphology with rSR in V1.

- Negative T waves from V1 to V3.

Incomplete RBBB

The appearance of the ECG is similar to that of complete RBBB but with QRS duration < 120 ms. Conduction is not blocked but only slowed [10].

Bi or Trifascicular Block

The most frequent form of bifascicular block is the combination of RBBB with a left anterior hemiblock (left axis deviation (between -30° and + 90°). Rarely RBBB is associated with left posterior hemiblock (right axis deviation (> +90°) (Figs. **19, 20** and **21**).

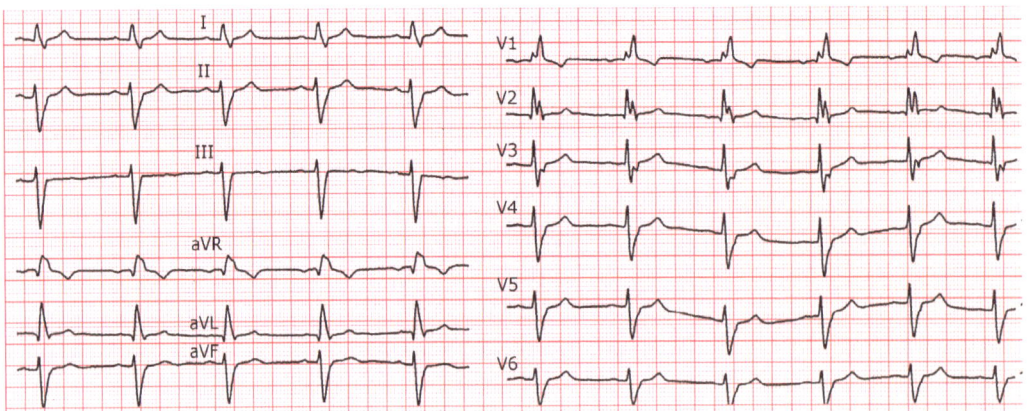

Figure 19: Sinus rhythm with RBBB and left anterior hemiblock.

The strict definition of trifascicular block is the combination of RBBB with alternating block in the 2 left hemibranches. Other types of bi- or trifascicular block cannot be diagnosed on the surface ECG a) simultaneous block in both left hemibranches (complete LBBB morphology) b) concomitant block in both branches of the His bundle, c) complete block in the right branch and of the 2 left hemibranches which causes complete A-V block.

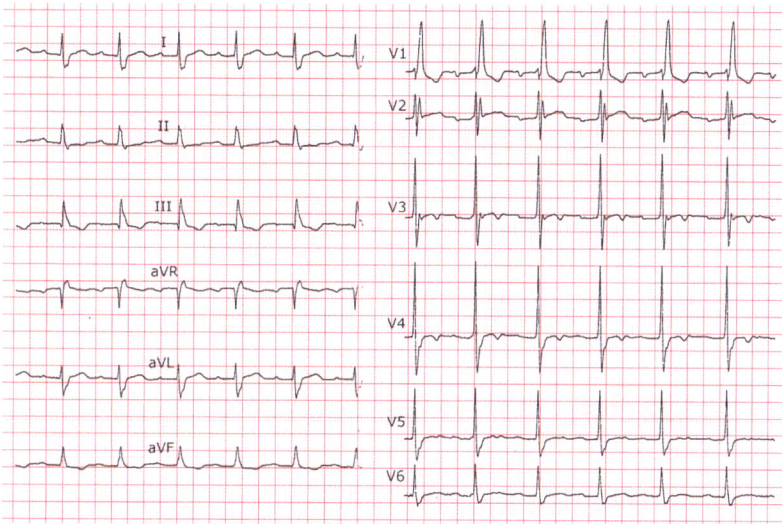

Figure 20: Sinus rhythm with RBBB and first degree A-V block.

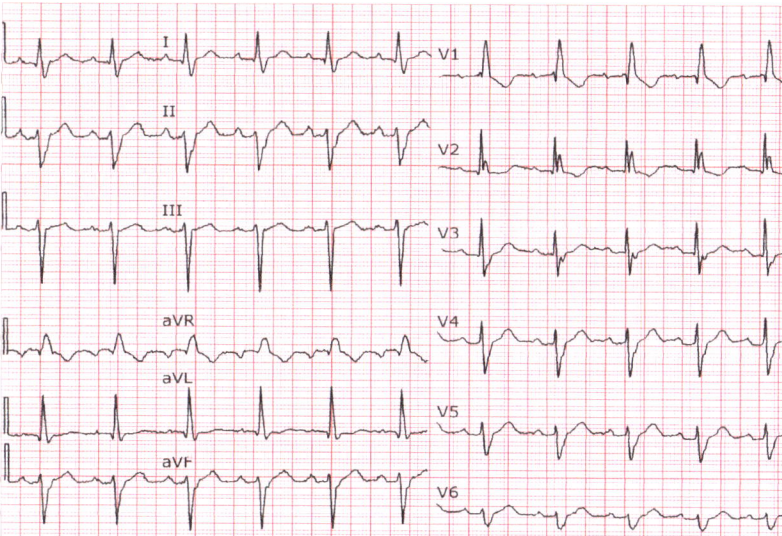

Figure 21: Sinus rhythm with RBBB, left anterior hemiblock and first degree A-V block.

SINO-ATRIAL BLOCK

First Degree Sino-Atrial Block

Sinus activity is not visible on the surface ECG. Thus, first degree sino-atrial block is only theoretical without electrophysiological sequelae. Only second and third degree sino-atrial block are visible on the surface ECG and these do have some clinical importance [3-6].

Second Degree Sino-Atrial Block

Second degree block of the type Wenckebach occurs with a progressive shortening of the PP interval and a slight increase of the heart rate followed by a pause with a duration greater than the PP interval preceding it but less than the next PP interval. Mobitz II second degree block can be diagnosed only if it is intermittent. Sinus pauses occur intermittently with their PP interval equal to exact multiples of the baseline PP interval. If the block is permanent, it only produces an apparent sinus bradycardia. For example, a permanent 2:1 sino-atrial block will simply halve the heart rate (Fig. **22**) [3-5].

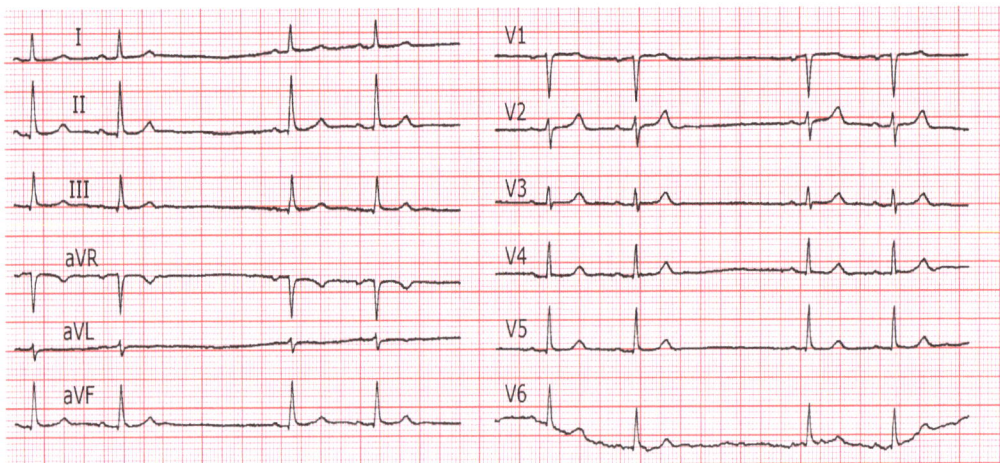

Figure 22: Second degree sino-atrial block with a pause exactly double that of the baseline PP interval.

Third Degree Sino-Atrial Block

Third degree block or complete block cannot be distinguished at all from true atrial standstill: absence of atrial activity, His bundle escape rhythm with narrow

QRS complexes and sometimes retrograde P' waves with a polarity opposite to sinus P wave polarity (Fig. **23**) [3-5].

When the sinus node fails to function for a significant period of time (sinus arrest), another part of the conduction system usually assumes the role of pacemaker. These pacing beats are referred to as escape beats and may come from the atria, the atrioventricular junction, or the ventricles. The pause can follow an episode of atrial tachyarrhythmia and is called tachy-brady syndrome (Fig. **24**).

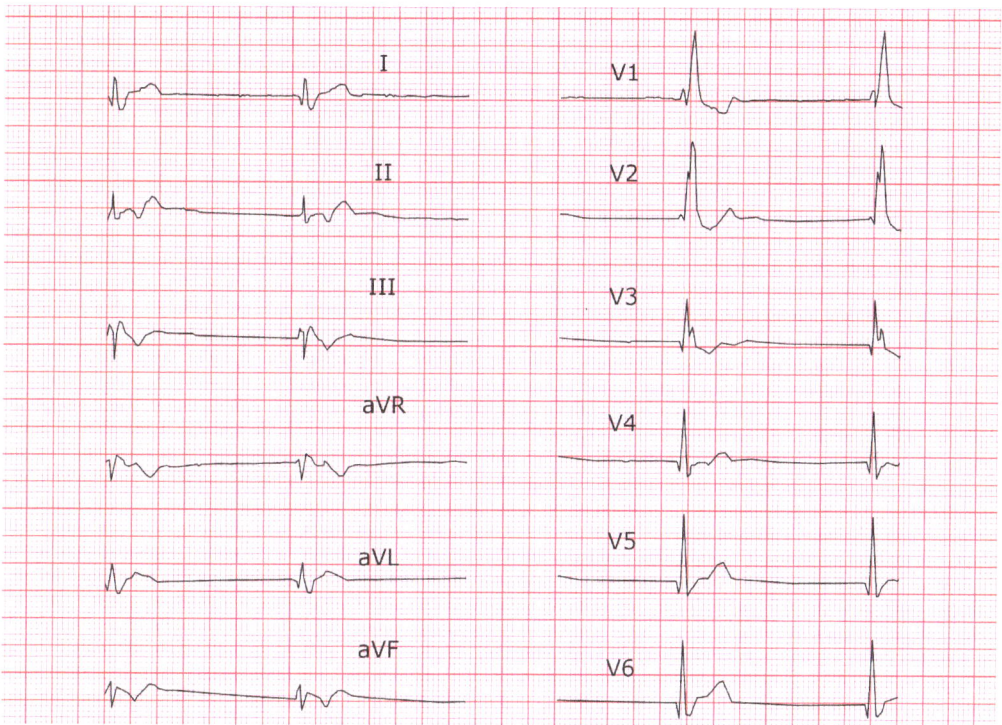

Figure 23: QRS complexes without P waves due to sinus arrest with nodal escape rhythm and conduction abnormalities (RBBB). Retrograde P' waves are visibles in the T wave (negative in II, III and aVF).

PACEMAKERS

The pacemaker rhythm can easily be recognized on the ECG. It shows pacemaker spikes: vertical artifact signals that represent the electrical activity of the pacemaker. Usually these spikes are more visible in unipolar than in bipolar pacing. The morphology of the QRS complex helps to locate the site of ventricular pacing, typically right bundle branch block morphology for left ventricular pacing and left bundle branch block morphology for right ventricular pacing. Pacemakers are categorized according to an international coding system that consists of 3-5 letters (Table **1**):

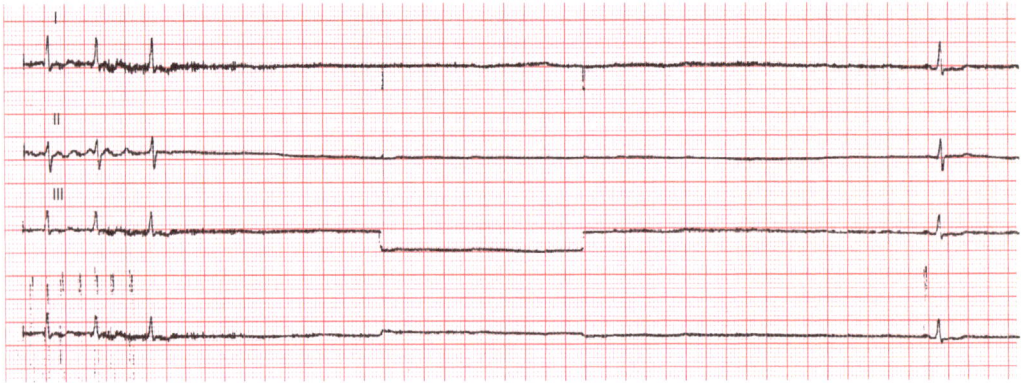

Figure 24: Atrial tachycardia on the left side of the trace followed by sinus arrest.

Table 1: The Revised NASPE/BPEG Generic Code for Antibradycardia Pacing

I	II	III	IV	V
Chamber(s) paced	Chamber(s) sensed	Response to sensing	Rate modulation	Multisite pacing
O = None	O = None	O = None	O = None	O = None
A = Atrium	A = Atrium	T = Triggered	R = Rate modulation	A = Atrium
V = Ventricle	V = Ventricle	I = Inhibited	V = Ventricle	
D = Dual (A+V)	D = Dual (A+V)	D = Dual (T+I)	D = Dual (A+V)	

Recently, new pacing modalities have been developed: Biventricular pacemakers (CRT-P): One ventricular lead is positioned in the right ventricle and the other at the surface of the left ventricle in a tributary vein of the coronary sinus in order to mechanically synchronize the ventricles. This cardiac resynchronization therapy can improve symptoms and survival in heart failure patients. The most effective interventricular pacing delay can be determined by means of non-invasive methods like echocardiography.

Combined with an ICD (Internal Cardioverter Defibrillator): This device detects and treats ventricular tachyarrhythmias. ICDs also have a pacing function. Usually the first treatment for ventricular arrhythmias is anti-tachy pacing (pacing at a rate

+/-10% above the ventricular rate in ventricular tachycardia) or ventricular cardioversion or defibrillation with a shock of 1-35 Joules of energy. All ICDs have optional pacing modalities to treat bradycardias. New biventricular ICDs have 3 leads: an atrial lead, a left ventricular lead and a right ventricular lead. They allowed resynchronization of cardiac activity. They are called biventricular ICDs (CRT-D): an ICD with biventricular pacing capacities.

Examples, of some of the most frequent electrocardiograms, in patients with pacemakers (Figs. **25** to **33**). Troubleshooting is not exhaustively presented because of the significant numbers and sometimes, extreme complexity.

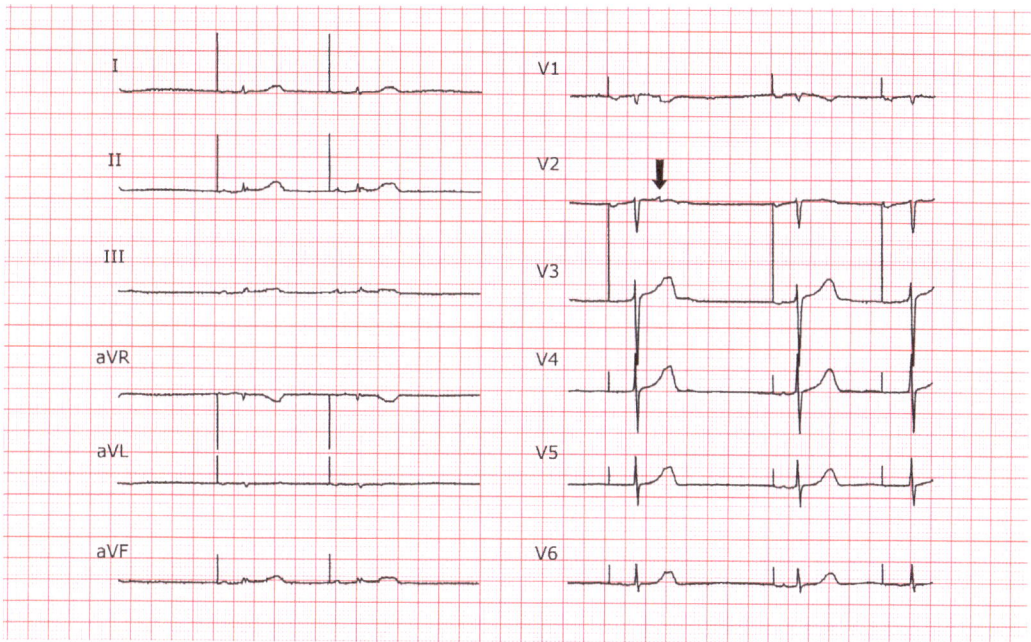

Figure 25: Atrial paced rhythm (AAI pacemaker). The size of the spike is typical for a unipolar system. The arrow shows a blocked P' wave which reset the pacemaker. The delay between the P' wave and the next spike is the escape rhythm of the pacemaker.

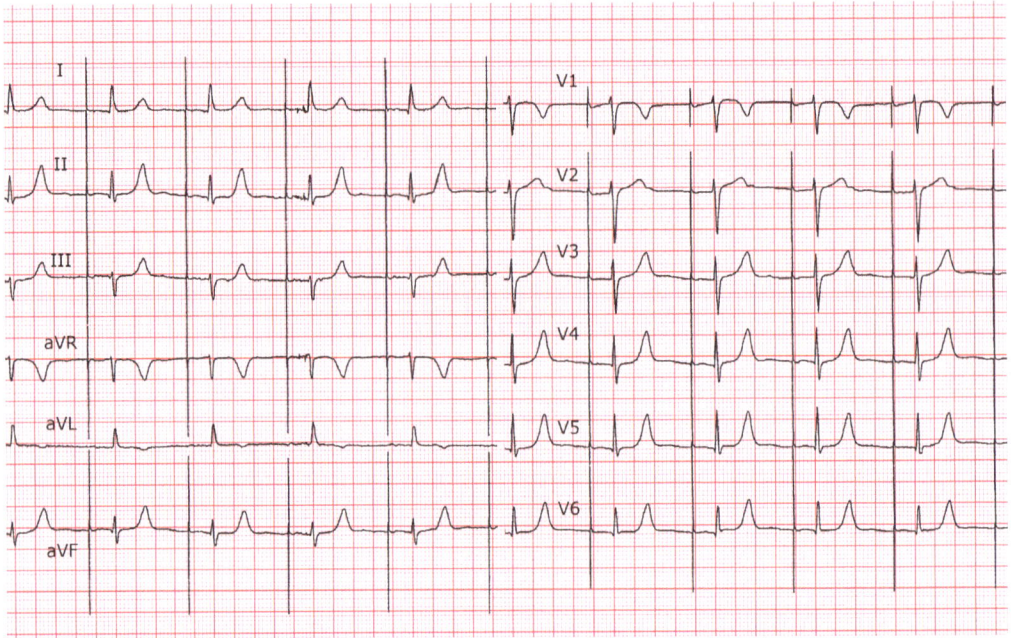

Figure 26: Another example of atrial paced rhythm in a patient with DDDR pacemaker. The device functions in a unipolar mode. The negative T wave is the sign of intermittent ventricular pacing (Chatterjee phenomenon).

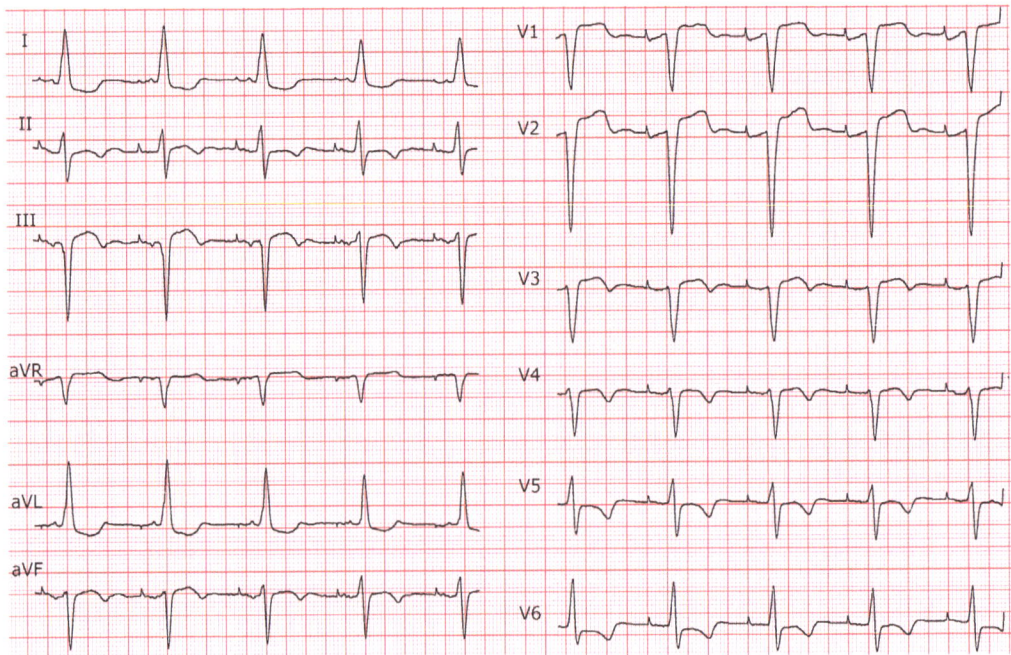

Figure 27: Atrial paced rhythm in a bipolar mode.

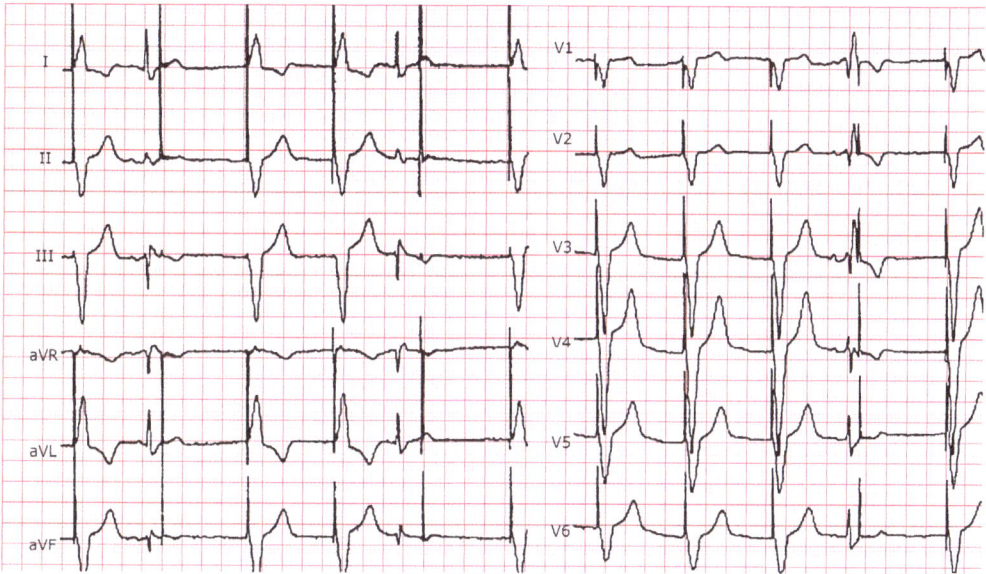

Figure 28: Ventricular paced rhythm (VVI pacemaker). The size of the spike is typical for a unipolar system. However the sensing function failed. The second complex from the left is a sinus beat, which should have been detected if the pacemaker was functionning correctly. The same default is present in V1 (QRS number 4). The pacing function is correct. The left bundle branch morphology of the QRS complex is typical for a pacemaker stimulating the right ventricular apex.

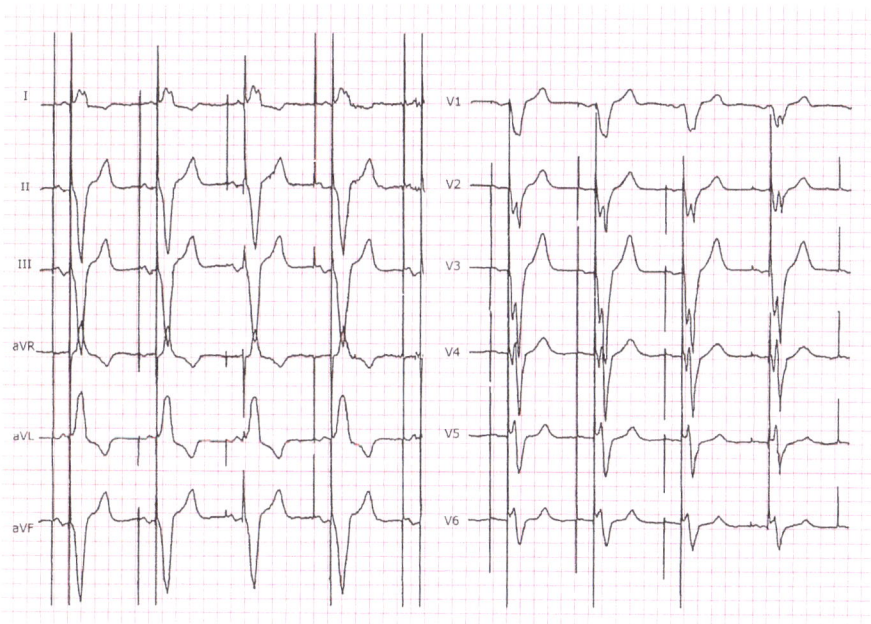

Figure 29: Atrial and ventricular paced rhythm (DDD pacemaker). The size of spike is typical for unipolar system in both chambers. Pacing is permanent in both chambers.

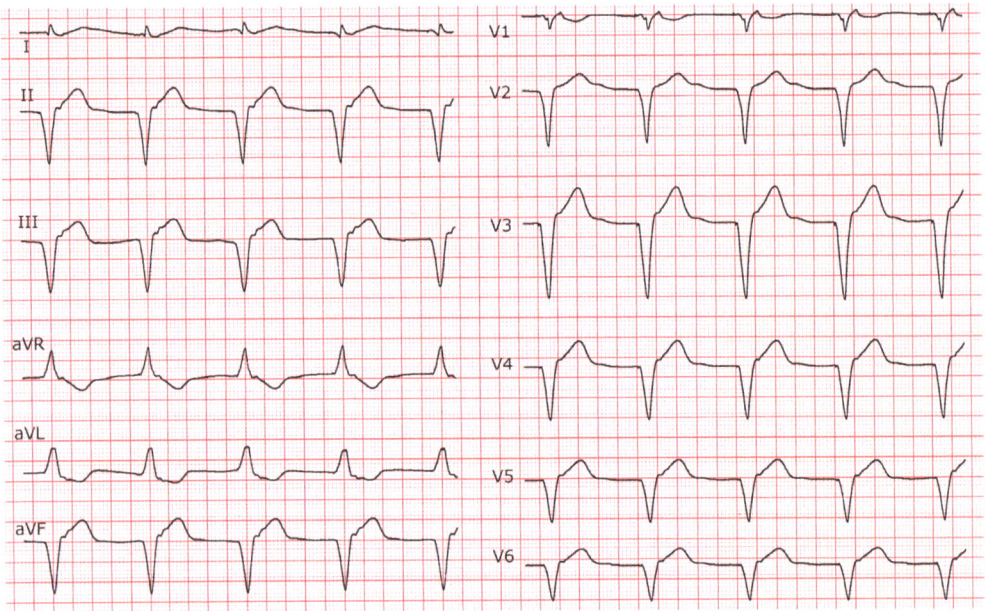

Figure 30: Permanent atrial and ventricular pacing in a patient with DDDR pacemaker. The spikes are visible in I (atrial spike) and in V3 and V4 (ventricular spike). The size of the spikes is very small because of a bipolar mode of stimulation.

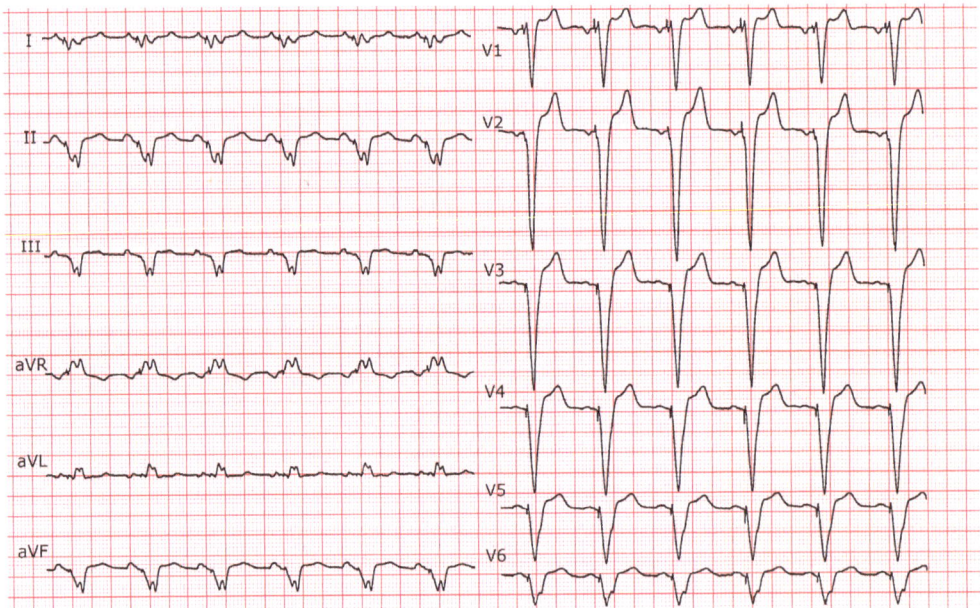

Figure 31: Spontaneous sinus activity followed by pacing of the right ventricle in a patient with DDDR pacemaker. The morphology of the QRS complex (left bundle branch block morphology) is typical for right ventricular pacing. The device functions in a bipolar mode.

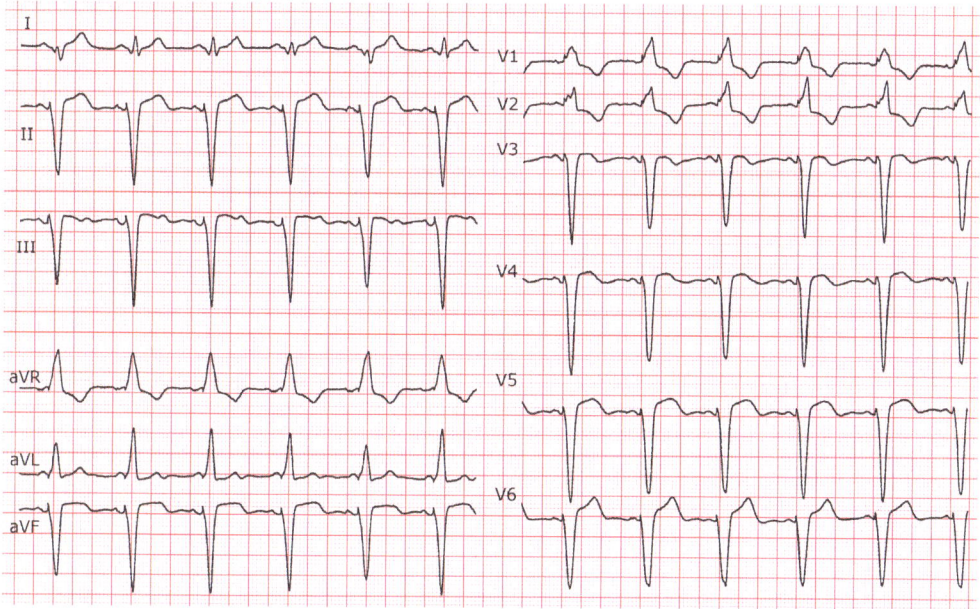

Figure 32: Spontaneous sinus activity followed by pacing of both ventricles in a patient with biventricular pacing (CRT-P). No spike can be seen before the P wave, although 2 spikes are present in the first part of the QRS complex. The morphology of the QRS complex in V1 (right bundle branch block morphology) is typical for biventricular pacing.

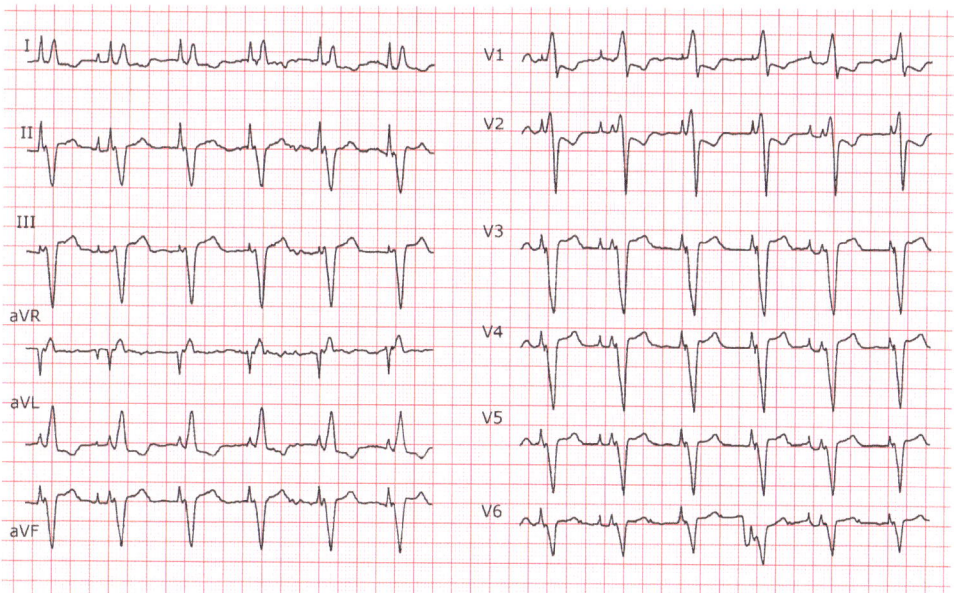

Figure 33: Atrial and biventricular pacing in a patient with CRT-P pacemaker. The device functions permanently in a bipolar mode. The morphology of the QRS complex is typical for biventricular pacing. Two spikes are visible in the initial part of the QRS complex.

ACKNOWLEDGEMENT

Declared none.

CONFLICT OF INTEREST

The author(s) confirm that this chapter content has no conflict of interest.

REFERENCES

[1]   Braunwald's Heart Disease : A Textbook of Cardiovascular Medicine: Elsevier- Saunders, 2011.

[2]   MacFarlane PW, Lawrie TDV (eds): Comprehensive Electrocardiology: Theory and Practice in Health and Disease. Vol 3. New York, Pergamon, 1989.

[3]   Kennedy HL, Goldberger AL, Graboys TB, et al: American College of Cardiology guidelines for training in adult cardiovascular medicine. Task Force 2: Training in electrocardiography, ambulatory electrocardiography, and exercise testing. J Am Coll Cardiol 25:1013, 1995.

[4]   Chou T-C, Knilans TK: Electrocardiography in Clinical Practice: Adult and Pediatric. 4th ed. Philadelphia, WB Saunders, 1996.

[5]   Schlant RC, Adolph RJ, DiMarco JP, et al: Guidelines for electrocardiography. A report of the American College of Cardiology/American Heart Association Task Force on Assessment of Diagnostic and Therapeutic Cardiovascular Procedures (Committee on Electrocardiography). Circulation 85:1221-1228,1992.
        MB, Elizari MV, Lazzari JO: The Hemiblocks. Oldsmar, FL, Tampa Tracings, 1970.

[6]   Selvester RH, Velasquez DW, Elko PP, Cady LD: Intraventricular conduction defect (IVCD), real or fancied: QRS duration in 1,254 normal adult white males by a multilead automated algorithm. J Electrocardiol 23(Suppl):118-122,

[7]   Parharidis G, Nouskas J, Efthimiadis G, et al: Complete left bundle branch block with left QRS axis deviation: Defining its clinical importance. Acta Cardiol 52:295-303, 1997.

[8]   Nikolic G, Marriott HJ: Left bundle branch block with right axis deviation: A marker of congestive cardiomyopathy. J Electrocardiol 18:395-404, 1985.

[9]   De Leonardis V, Goldstein SA, Lindsay J Jr: Electrocardiographic diagnosis of left ventricular hypertrophy in the presence of complete right bundle branch block. Am J Cardiol 62:590-593, 1988.

[10]   Spodick DH: Fascicular blocks: Not interpretable from the electrocardiogram. Am J Cardiol 70:809-810, 1992.

[11]   Hancock EW, Deal BJ, Mirvis DM, Okin P, Kligfield P, Gettes LS. Recommendations for the Standardization and Interpretation of the Electrocardiogram. Circulation 2009; 119: e251-e261.

Send Orders of Reprints at reprints@benthamscience.net

Electrocardiography (ECG), 2013, 53-99

CHAPTER 4

Arrhythmias and Tachycardias

Abstract: In this chapter, we address the basic notions of cardiac arrhythmias. Premature ventricular and atrial contractions, also known as "extrasystoles", are "extra" heartbeats. Atrial premature beats, describes premature beats arising from the atrium. Ectopic P' wave morphology differs from sinus beats and varies depending on the origin of the premature beat. The mechanism of the tachycardia is macro-reentry or automaticity \and the rate varies between 140 and 220 bpm. There are two types of atrial flutter, the common type I and the rarer type II. Most individuals with atrial flutter will manifest only one of these. Rarely someone may manifest both types. Flutter originates either from the right or left atrium depending on its cause. Typical atrial flutter (90% of cases) is caused by a macro re-entry in the right atrium, with a regular rate of about 300 beats per minute. Atrial fibrillation is a consequence of multiple atrial micro reentry circuits. The arrhythmia is described as irregularly irregular because of the complete disorganization of the atrial electrical activity. Characteristic findings are the absence of P waves, with unorganized electrical activity in their place ("f" waves), at a rate of 350 to 500/minute and irregularity of the R-R interval due to irregular conduction of impulses to the ventricles.

AV nodal reentrant tachycardia (AVNRT) is also called junctional tachycardia. AVNRT is usually a reentrant tachycardia using a reentry circuit located within the AV node area. In the typical form of AVNRT (> 90% of the cases), the reentry circuit uses the slow pathway antegradely and the fast pathway retrogradely. Antegrade ventricular activation occurs simultaneously with the retrograde atrial activation. The P' wave is hidden in the QRS complex, sometimes visible as a small r' wave in V1 at the end of the QRS complex. Rarely it can be seen as a small q wave in the inferior leads. Comparison of the trace in tachycardia and in sinus rhythm facilitates the diagnosis unless conduction abnormalities (BBB) are present during tachycardia. In the atypical form (5-10%of cases), the reentry circuit uses the fast pathway antegradely and the slow pathway retrogradely. The P' wave is negative in the inferior leads with a ratio P'R/RP'< 1 as in atrial tachycardia from which it should be differentiated. In the normal heart, electrical signals use only one pathway to propagate through the heart. This is the atrio-ventricular or A-V node.

If there is an extra conduction pathway present, the electrical signal may arrive at the ventricle too soon. This condition is called Wolff-Parkinson-White syndrome (WPW). It is in a category of electrical abnormalities called "pre-excitation syndromes". The electrical properties of this pathway, which is basically an abnormal muscular connection between the atrium and the ventricle, are different from those of the normal A-V conduction system and creates the conditions for a reentry circuit. The accessory pathway can conduct exclusively antegradely, in other words from the atrium to the ventricle, exclusively retrogradely, from the ventricle to the atrium or in a bidirectional manner. It can be located anywhere in the A-V groove but predominantely in the lateral

Jean-Jacques Goy, Jean-Christophe Stauffer, Jürg Schlaepfer and Pierre Christeler

region. Orthodromic tachycardia is the most common arrhythmia associated with accessory pathways. It is a macro-reentry circuit using the A-V node antegradely and the accesory pathway retrogradely. Passage through this accessory pathway delays the retrograde activation of the atrium. This manifests, on the ECG, as a time delay between the QRS complex and the next P' wave (> 100 ms). Less commonly, a shorter refractory period in the accessory tract may cause block of an ectopic atrial impulse in the normal A-V pathway, with antegrade conduction down the accessory tract and then retrograde conduction up the normal (A-V) pathway. This type of tachycardia produced is called antidromic tachycardia. The QRS complex is wide (> 140 ms), with an exaggeration of the delta wave seen during sinus rhythm (wide-QRS tachycardia). Atrial fibrillation is the third arrhythmia occuring in patients with accessory pathways. The depolarisation can reach the ventricles by both the normal A-V pathway and the accessory pathway. If the latter has a short refractory period and as conduction can be very fast over this accessory pathway, the ventricular response can be very high, up to 300 bpm and irregular. The QRS complexes are wide but with a variable width depending on the use of the accessory pathway by the depolarisation. Permanent junctional re-entrant tachycardia is a relatively uncommon form of re-entry tachycardia with antegrade conduction occurring through the atrioventricular node and retrograde conduction over an accessory pathway usually located in the postero-septal region. It is a macroreentry circuit using the A-V node antegradely and the accessory pathway retrogradely. The P' wave is negative in the limb leads with RP'>P'R.

Three or more beats that originate from the ventricle at a rate of more than 100 beats per minute constitute a ventricular tachycardia. If the fast rhythm self-terminates within 30 seconds, it is considered a non-sustained ventricular tachycardia. If the rhythm lasts more than 30 seconds it is known as a sustained ventricular tachycardia (even if it terminates on its own after 30 seconds). Ventricular tachycardia can be classified based on its morphology: monomorphic ventricular tachycardia means that the appearance of all the beats matches each other in each lead of a surface electrocardiogram. Polymorphic ventricular tachycardia, on the other hand, has beat-to-beat variation in morphology. The most common cause of monomorphic ventricular tachycardia is damaged or dead (scar) tissue from a previous myocardial infarction.

Ventricular fibrillation is a condition in which there is a fast un-coordinated contraction of the cardiac muscle of the ventricles in the heart. It is a chaotic dysynchronous activity of the heart without identifiable QRS complexes. If the arrhythmia continues for more than a few seconds, blood circulation will cease, and death will occur in a matter of minutes.

Keywords: Atrial extrasystoles, ventricular extrasystoles, supraventricular tachycardia, ventricular tachycardia, atrial tachycardia, atrioventriuclar tachycardia, Permanent Junctional Reentrant tachycardia, torsades de pointes, ventricular fibrillation, idioventricular accelerated rhythm, atrial tachycardia.

ACTION POTENTIAL

The cardiac action potential is a specialized action potential in the heart recorded inside the myocardial cell, with unique properties necessary for function of the electrical conduction system of the heart. Its activity depends on sodium, calcium, potassium and magnesium ion movements through the cell's membrane. This action potential has 5 phases as described in Chapter 1 [1, 2].

Important Concepts

- Excitability it depends on the metabolic state of the myocardial cell, on the depolarisation threshold, on the refractory periods of the tissue and on its inhomogeneity.

- Conduction. It is closely related to excitability since a cell can correctly transmit a depolarisation only when normally excitable. Moreover, the speed of depolarisation (phase 0) determines the conduction velocity.

- Automaticity. In the myocardium, automaticity is the ability of the cardiac muscles to depolarize spontaneously, without external electrical stimulation from the nervous system. This spontaneous depolarisation is due to the plasma membranes within the heart, which have reduced permeability to potassium but still allow passive transfer of sodium ions, allowing a net charge to build up. Automaticity is most often demonstrated in the sinoatrial node, the so-called "Pacemaker of the Heart" but can exist in all cardiac tissues. Abnormalities in automaticity result in rhythm changes.

Mechanism of Arrhythmias

1. Impulse impairment:

   - Abnormal automaticity. In abnormal automaticity, the rate of phase 4 depolarisation, may be slowed or increased. A tachycardia would result if the rate of phase 4 depolarisation increased. Arrhythmias caused by abnormal automaticity usually show gradual acceleration and deceleration (warm-up and cool-down phenomena).

- Triggered activity. Triggered activity occurs when abnormalities of the action potential cause one action potential to prematurely "trigger" another. In contrast to automaticity, this does not occur spontaneously. The most common abnormality of the action potential resulting in triggered activity is the presence of prolonged repolarisation. In triggered automaticity, the resting membrane potential and phase 4 depolarisation are normal but the repolarisation process of the action potential is interrupted by abnormal depolarisations, because they occur after the initial depolarisation they are called "after depolarisations" which may reach threshold and cause a second action potential. This can result in tachycardia often induced by drugs.

2. Conduction abnormalities. They are involved in the reentry mechanism. Three conditions are required for reentry:

- Localized conduction abnormality.

- Two separate anatomical pathways, one antegrade and one retrograde with different electrophysiological properties.

- Unidirectional block in one of the 2 pathways.

The following events are required for reentrant tachycardia induction [1-4] (Fig. **1**):

In sinus rhythm, the depolarisation uses the 2 pathways antegradely α and β. Conduction is faster over the α pathway than over the β one. When depolarisation reaches distal β nothing happens, the tissue, already having been depolarized by the fast pathway α is refractory. When atrial premature beats occur when the œ is refractoy (the refractory period of the α pathway is longer than that of the β pathway), depolarisation uses the slow pathway β, which is still excitable. Distally, depolarisation will continue downstream as well as retrogradely through the α pathway, which has not been used antegradely. Arriving back at the origin of the circuit, depolarisation can reactivate the β pathway no longer refractory. Circus movement tachycardia is induced. The mechansim of atrio-ventricular tachycardia using an accessory pathway and that of ventricular tachycardia is also reentry [1-4].

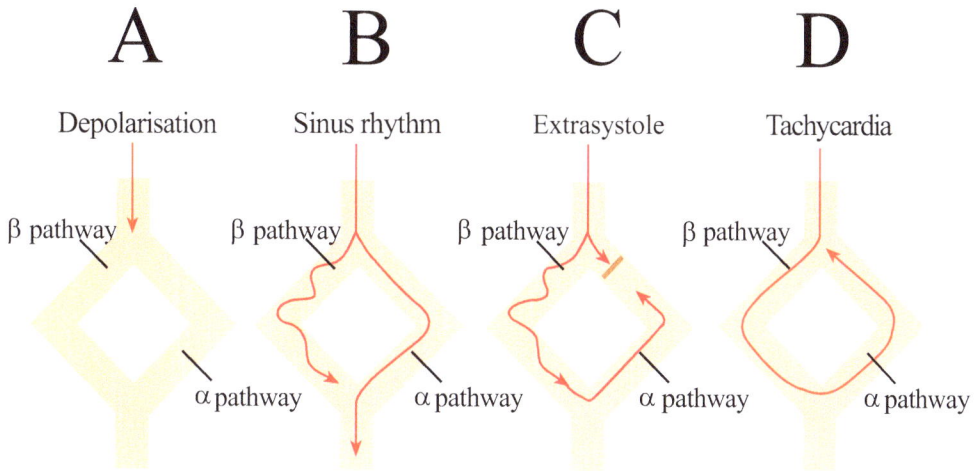

A   B   C   D

Depolarisation   Sinus rhythm   Extrasystole   Tachycardia

β pathway   β pathway   β pathway   β pathway

α pathway   α pathway   α pathway   α pathway

A
α Rapid conduction and long refractory period.
β Slow conduction and long refractory period.

B
α Depolarisation reaches the distal portion first and depolarises the tissue distally.
β The depolarisation is blocked in the distal portion of the pathway.

C
α Depolarisation is blocked in the initial portion of the α pathway.
β Depolarisation uses the βpathway antegradely and the α pathway retrogradely.

D
Tachycardia has been initiated.

Figure 1: Reentry phenomenon.

Prognosis and significance of tachycardias are related to the clinical situation. Patient management depends on the type and mechanism of the arrhythmia. It is useful to separate tachycardias based on QRS complex duration. Narrow QRS complex tachycardias (QRS duration < 120 ms) usually have a supraventricular origin, and wide QRS complex tachycardias (QRS duration > 120 ms), usually originate from the ventricles. Aberrant conduction or preexcited tachycardias are the exception. Tachycardias associated with the Wolff-Parkinson-White syndrome constitute a special case exhibiting wide or narrow QRS depending on the electrophysiological conditions.

EXTRASYSTOLES

Premature ventricular and atrial contractions, also known as "extrasystoles", are "extra" heartbeats. They arise from an irritable area in the heart. Extrasystoles interrupt the normal heart rhythm and cause an irregular beat. The mechanism of extrasystoles is, either enhanced automaticity (post-depolarisation), triggered activity or reentry. Extrasystoles may originate from the atria, the ventricles or the A-V node, each manifesting a different but characteristic electrocardiographic morphology. Extrasystoles are distinguished by 2 criteria: their morphology and time course in the cardiac cycle [1, 3, 5].

Atrial Premature Beats

Atrial premature beats, describes premature beats arising from the atrium. Ectopic P' wave morphology differs from sinus beats and varies depending on the origin of the premature beat (Fig. **2**).

Premature beats originating from the sinus node region have almost the same appearance as normal sinus P waves. Those originating from the low right atrium are negative in the inferior limb leads II, III, aVF. Those originating from the mid-atrium are biphasic (Fig. **3**) and finally those originating from the left atrium are negative in limb leads I and aVL (Figs. **3** and **4**).

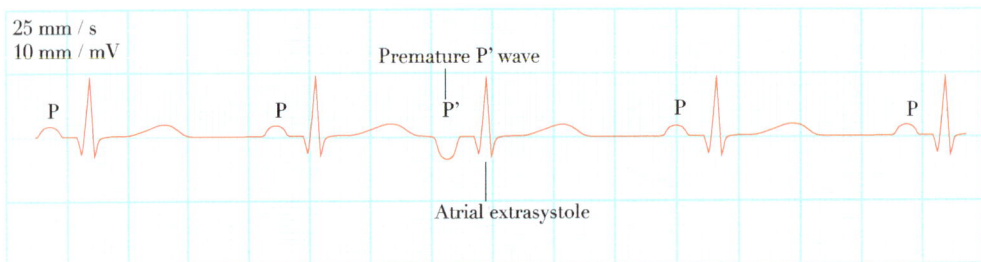

Figure 2: Atrial premature beat with P' wave.

Depending on the prematurity of the atrial impulse and refractoriness of the A-V node and conduction system, the P wave may conduct with normal or prolonged PR interval, with narrow or aberrant QRS complexes (bundle branch block) or may block and not be followed by a QRS complex (Fig. **4**). In this case a pause is seen on the trace because of retrograde depolarisation of the sinus node and resetting (Figs. **5**, **6** and **7**).

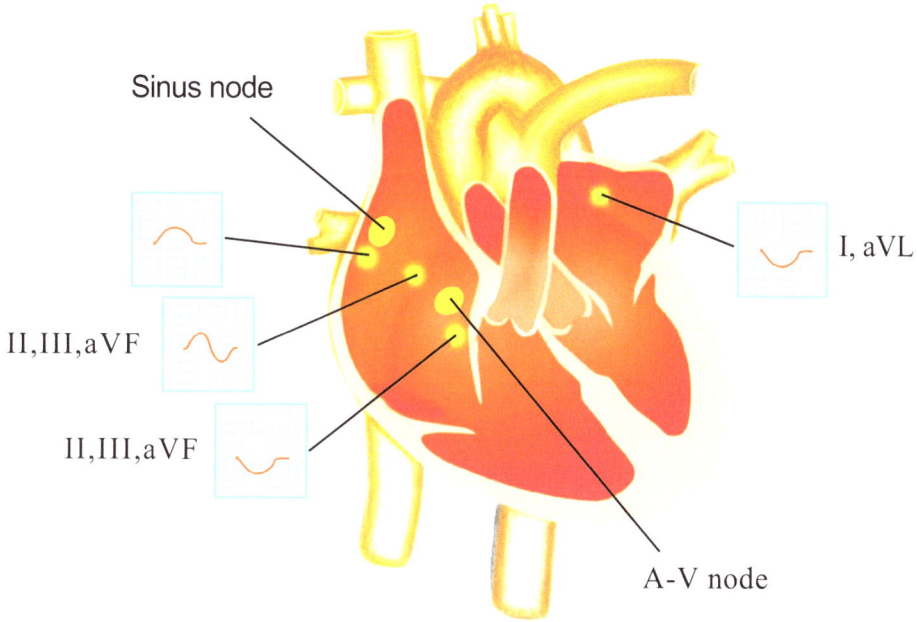

Figure 3: Atrial premature beats: P' wave is: negative in limb leads I and aVL when the premature beat arises from the left atrium, biphasic when originating from the mid right atrium and negative in limb leads II, III and aVL when originating from the low right atrium.

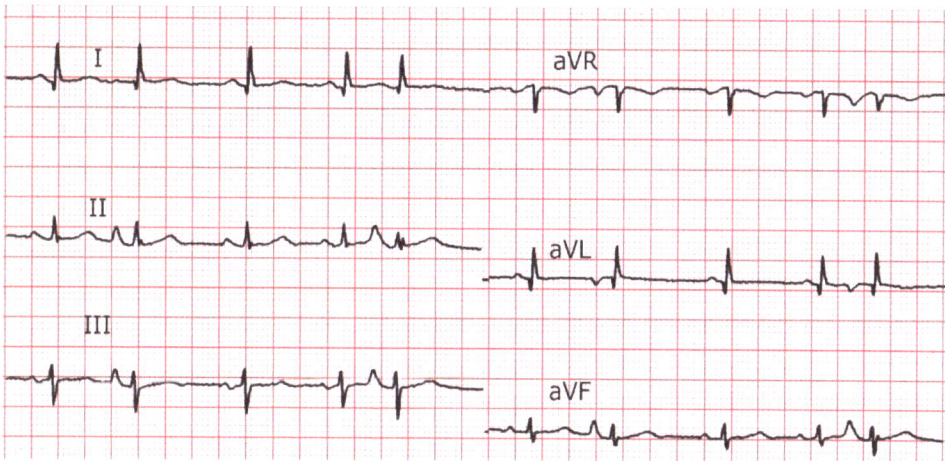

Figure 4: Left atrial premature beats. (Negative P' waves in I and aVL). The P' wave modifies the T wave and the PR interval is prolonged because of the slowing of the impulse in the A-V node. The following QRS complex is slightly different because of some conduction abnormalities in the His-Purkinje system.

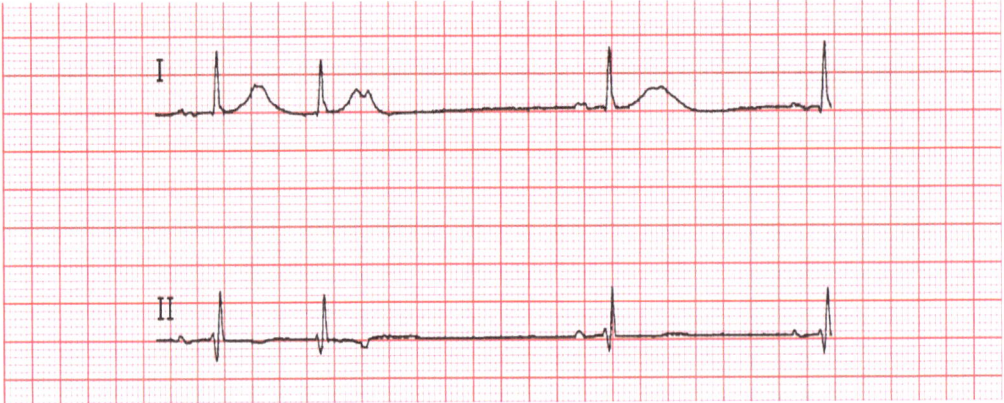

Figure 5: The first complex on the left originates from the sinus node. It is followed by 2 atrial premature beats, one with a long PR interval and the second blocked.

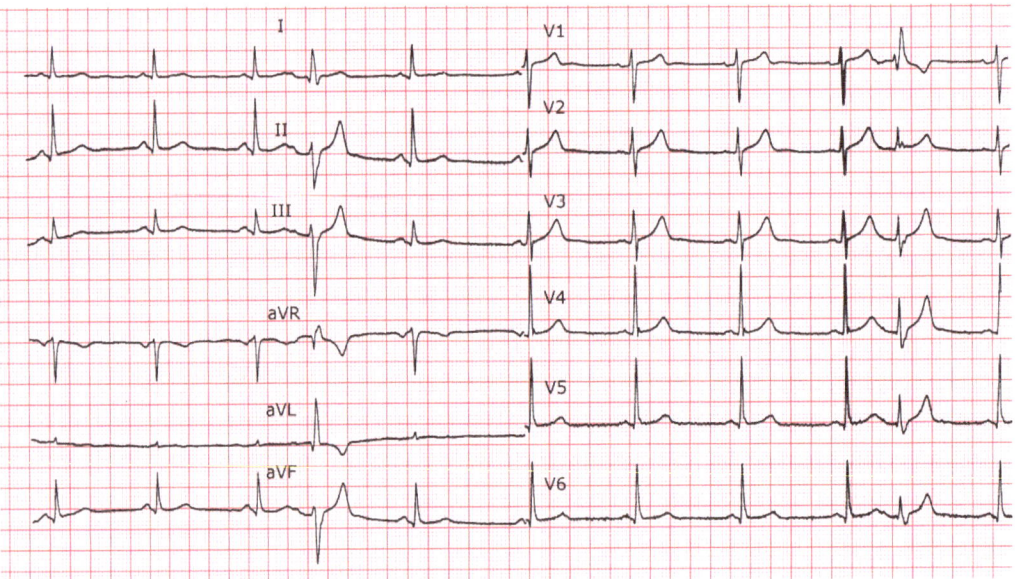

Figure 6: Sinus rhythm at 60 bpm. The second beat from the left is a right atrial premature beat with aberrant conduction and left anterior hemiblock and prolonged PR interval. The penultimate complex is another atrial premature beat with a RBBB aberration.

Ventricular Premature Contractions

They arise from an irritable area in the ventricles, interrupt the normal heart rhythm and cause an irregular beat. Conduction is slow and the QRS complex is wide (>120 ms). Its morphology varies greatly and depends on its site of origin [1-4] (Fig. **8**).

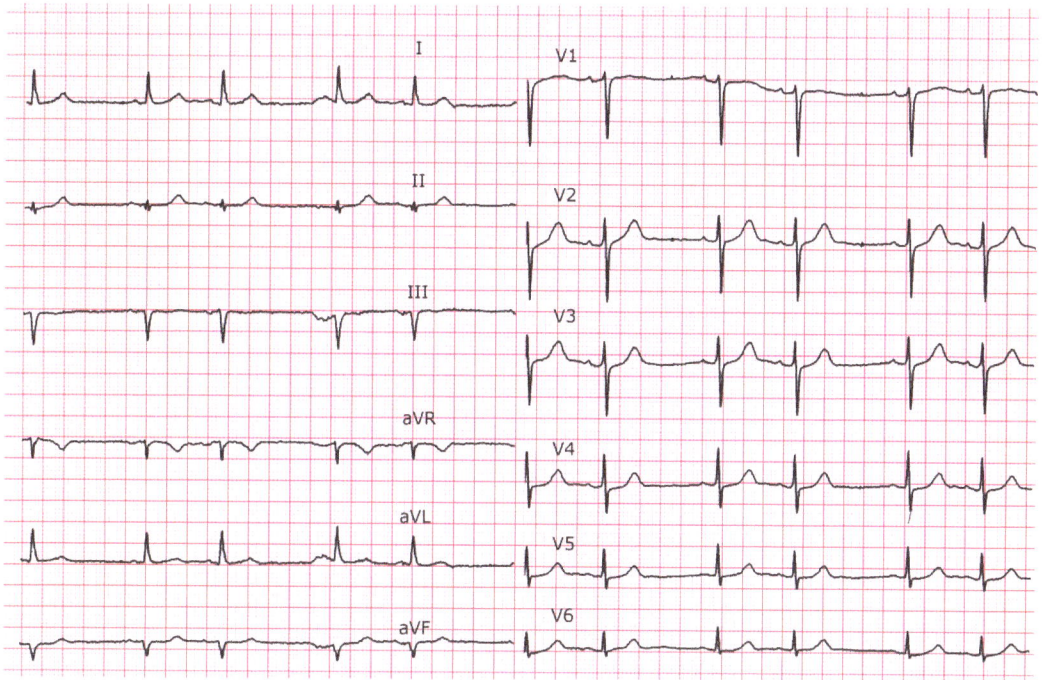

Figure 7: Bigeminy of right atrial premature beats.

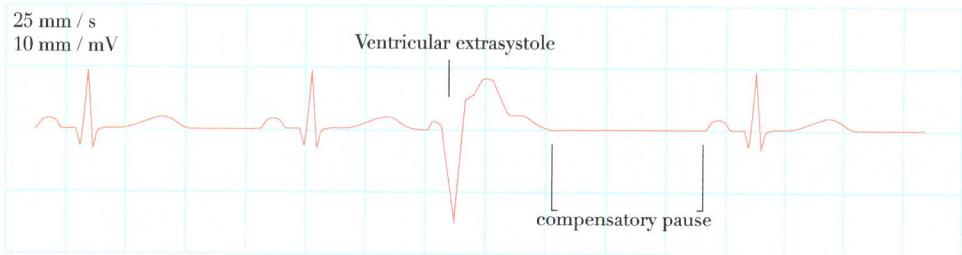

Figure 8: Ventricular extrasystoles.

A left ventricular premature contraction activates first the left ventricle, then the septum and finally the right ventricle. This is somewhat similar to right bundle activation. Thus the QRS complex of these ventricular premature contractions has some similarity to the QRS complex of RBBB (predominant r wave in V1). Similarly, ventricular premature contractions arising from the right ventricle resemble the QRS complex of LBBB (deep S wave in V1).

Ventricular extrasystoles with right axis deviation and left bundle branch morphology in the precordial leads arise from the pulmonary outflow tract. They are usually benign unless associated with right ventricular dysplasia. However, multifocal ventricular extrasystoles are, in principle associated with cardiomyopathies, often, ischemic heart disease. Usually, premature ventricular contractions are followed by a "compensatory pause". This means that the interval between the QRS preceding the premature ventricular contraction and the one following it is double that of the baseline RR interval and that the premature ventricular contraction does not interfere with the baseline sinus rhythm.

In some cases, the abnormal wave of depolarisation will also travel through the conduction system in a retrograde fashion, and depolarize the atria and sinus node as well, allowing repolarisation to occur sooner. This results in an incomplete compensatory pause and the interval between the last normal QRS and the next normal QRS will be less than twice the average RR interval. In some cases, the premature ventricular contraction does not affect the atria at all, and the next P wave and normal QRS occur as if the PVC was not present, and there is no compensatory pause. These types of PVC are called interpolated premature ventricular contractions.

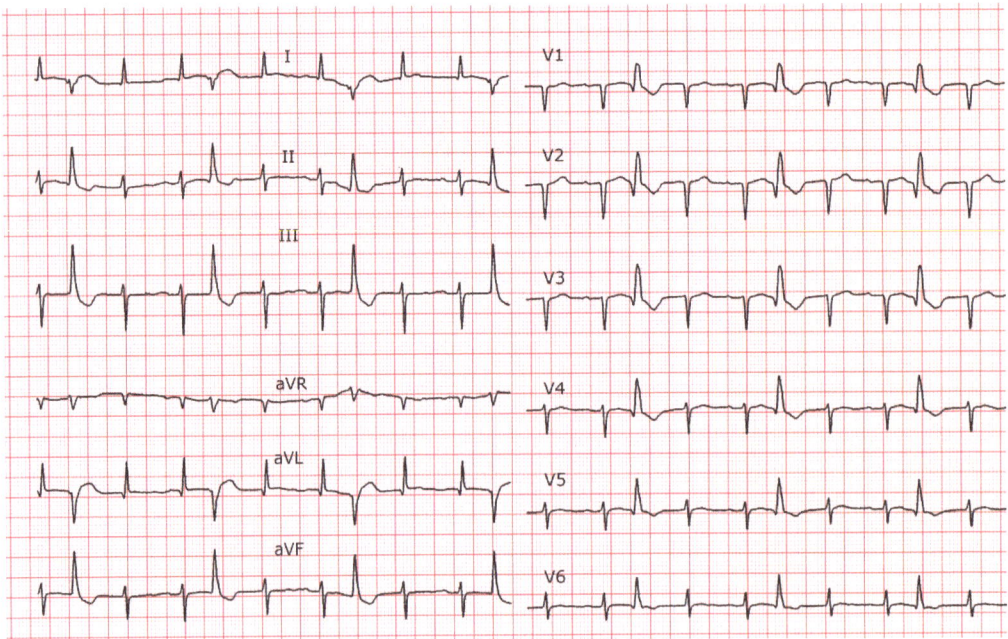

Figure 9: Trigeminism of ventricular premature contractions with right axis deviation and RBBB morphology.

Premature ventricular contraction may occur at regular intervals. If a premature ventricular contraction occurs after every normal QRS, this is termed ventricular bigeminy. If it occurs after every two normal QRS complexes, this is termed ventricular trigeminy (Fig. **9**). Doublets is defined as 2 consecutive ventricular premature contractions. Three consecutive ventricular premature contractions already represent a salvo of non-sustained ventricular tachycardia (Figs. **10** and **11**).

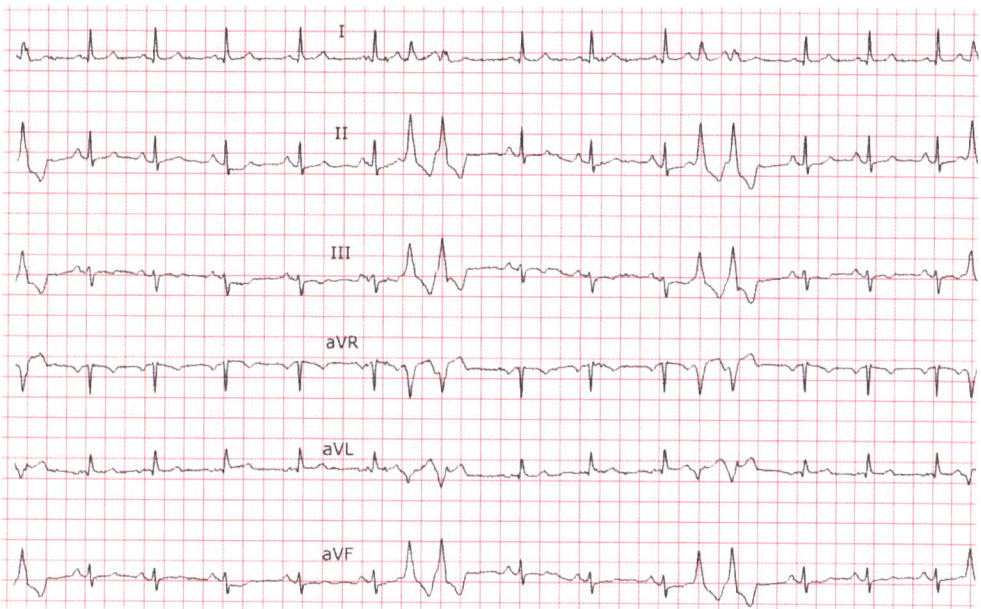

Figure 10: Ventricular premature contractions in doublets with right axis deviation arising from the right ventricular outflow tract.

SUPRAVENTRICULAR TACHYCARDIA

Tachycardia should be separated into 2 groups: the narrow QRS complex tachycardia which is usually supraventricular tachycardia and the wide QRS complex tachycardia which usually implies ventricular tachycardia or supraventricular tachycardia mimicking ventricular tachycardia because of aberrant conduction.

Atrial Tachycardia

The mechanism of the tachycardia is macro-reentry or automaticity \and the rate varies between 140 and 220 bpm. When different P waves (at least 3 morphologies) are present, the tachycardia is called multifocal atrial tachycardia or wandering pacemaker. This tachycardia often precedes atrial fibrillation. The P' wave morphology depends on the origin of the impulse in the atrium.

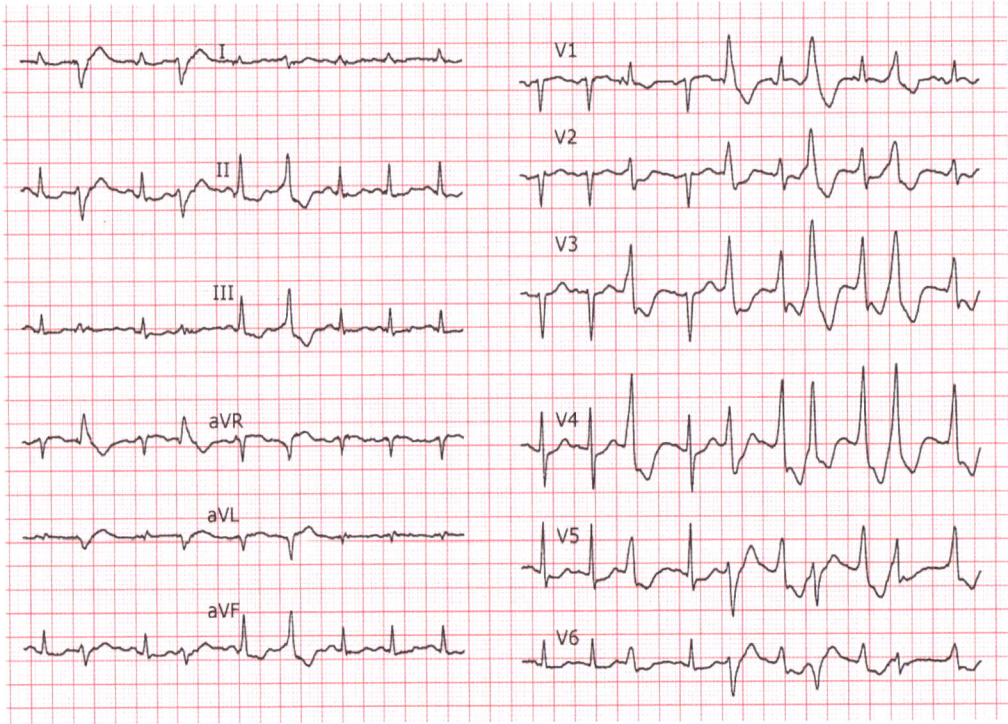

Figure 11: Polymorphic ventricular premature contractions, with bigeminy and brief salvos of ventricular tachycardia.

In tachycardia, the A-V conduction is usually 1:1, with one P' wave for each QRS complex. The conducted ventricular rhythm is also usually regular but may become irregular, often at higher atrial rates because of variable conduction through the A-V node, thus producing conduction patterns such as 2:1, 3:1, and Wenckebach A-V block. The P' wave is distant from the QRS complex with an RP' interval longer than the P'R interval (RP' > P'R or RP'/ P'R > 1) (Fig. **12**). The QRS complex is narrow unless a preexisting aberrant conduction is present. Second degree A-V block is obtained by, carotid sinus massage, "vagal maneuver" (carotid sinus compression, Valsalva maneuver) or drugs like verapamil, adenosine, beta-blockers or digitalis. Atrioventricular block facilitates the diagnosis (See Fig. **14**).

Carotid sinus massage helps in the differential diagnosis of tachycardias. It allows:

1.   Termination of AV nodal or orthodromic A-V tachycardia by blocking the impulse in the A-V node.

2.   Diagnosis of atrial flutter or atrial tachycardia by uncovering P' waves not followed with a QRS complex.

QRS morphology is normal unless a preexisting BBB is present. Functional BBB is related to high heart rate.

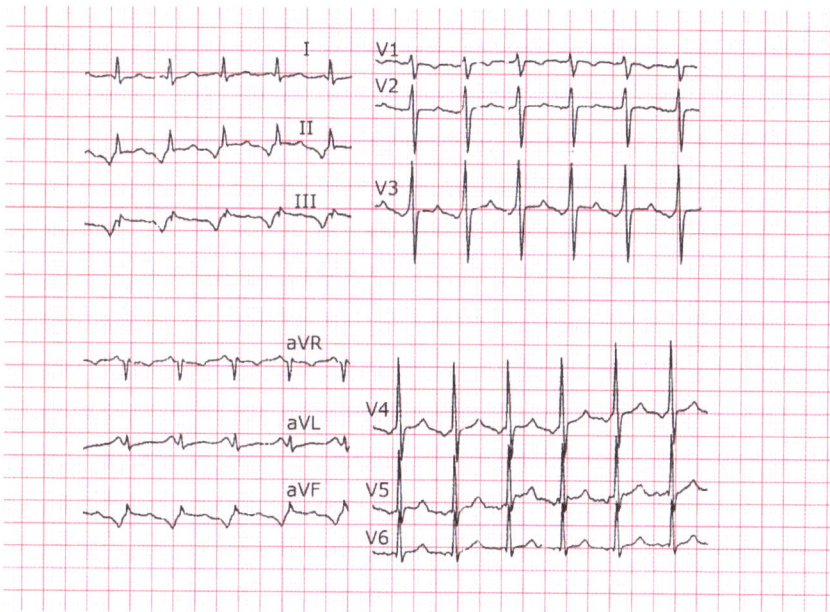

Figure 12: Atrial tachycadia with negative P' waves in limb leads II, III and aVF (RP'/P'R > 1) arising from the inferior right atrium.

Atrial Flutter

There are two types of atrial flutter, the common type I and the rare type II. Most individuals with atrial flutter will manifest only one of these. Rarely someone may manifest both types. Flutter originates either from the right or left atrium depending on its cause. Typical atrial flutter (90% of cases) is caused by a macro re-entry in the right atrium, with a regular rate of about 300 beats per minute (Fig. **13**). The reentrant loop forms a circuit in the right atrium, passing through the isthmus - a body of fibrous tissue in the lower atrium between the inferior vena cava and the tricuspid valve. The flutter waves "F" in this rhythm, are inverted in limb leads II, III, and aVF in the counterclockwise flutter (type I). The re-entry loop cycles are in the opposite direction in clockwise atrial flutter (typeII), thus the flutter waves are upright in II, III, and aVF. The flutter waves are called sawtooth waves; they are positive in V1, and negative in V6 (Fig. **13** and **14**). When different from this morphology the flutter is called « atypical » [1-4] (Fig. **15**).

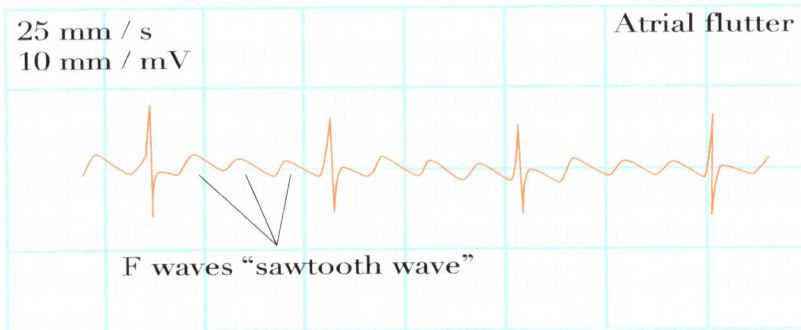

Figure 13: Typical atrial flutter.

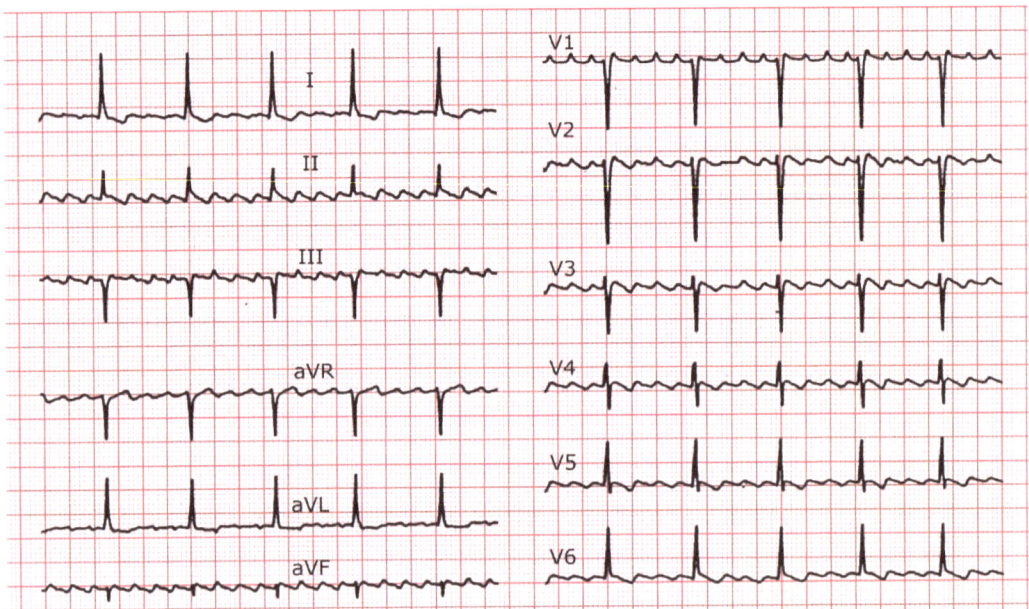

Figure 14: Typical atrial flutter with 4:1 A-V conduction. Ventricular rate is 75 bpm.

The rate of the flutter (F) waves is between 240 and 350 bpm. The rate of the QRS complexes depends on the conduction velocity of the A-V node, usually 150 bpm where one in two F waves is conducted to the ventricle. More rarely, the rate is 100 or 75 bpm especially in patients on antiarrhythmic drugs. The QRS complex is narrow unless there are conduction abnormalities associated with the flutter. Atrial flutter should always be considered as a possible diagnosis when the heart rate is 150 bpm. Vagal maneuvers allow an unmasking of the F waves.

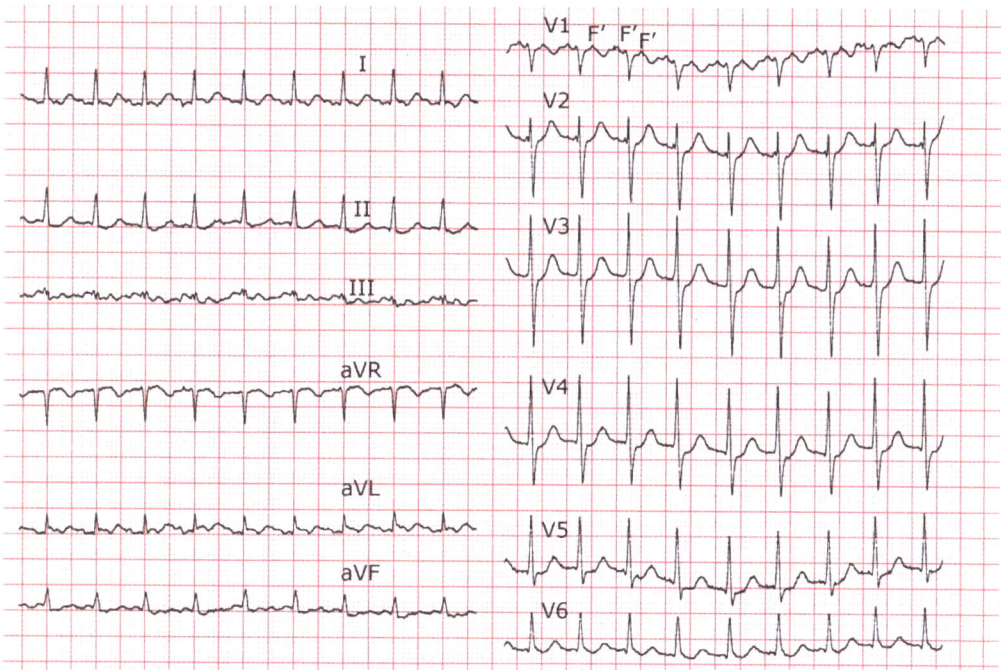

Figure 15: Atypical atrial flutter with 2:1 conduction. Flutter waves are best seen in V1 with a small F' wave in the T wave at the end of the QRS complex before the following QRS complex.

Atrial Fibrillation (AF)

Atrial fibrillation is a consequence of multiple atrial microreentry circuits. The arrhythmia is described as irregularly irregular because of the complete disorganization of the atrial electrical activity [1, 6]. Characteristic findings are the absence of P waves, with unorganized electrical activity in their place ("f" waves), at a rate of 350 to 500/minute and irregularity of the R-R interval due to irregular conduction of impulses to the ventricles. Most of the "f" waves are blocked in the A-V node, which acts as a gatekeeper avoiding high ventricular rate. A-V node conduction is random and ventricular rate is completely irregular (Figs. **16** and **17**). AF can be intermittent as is often seen in the focal type (Fig. **18**).

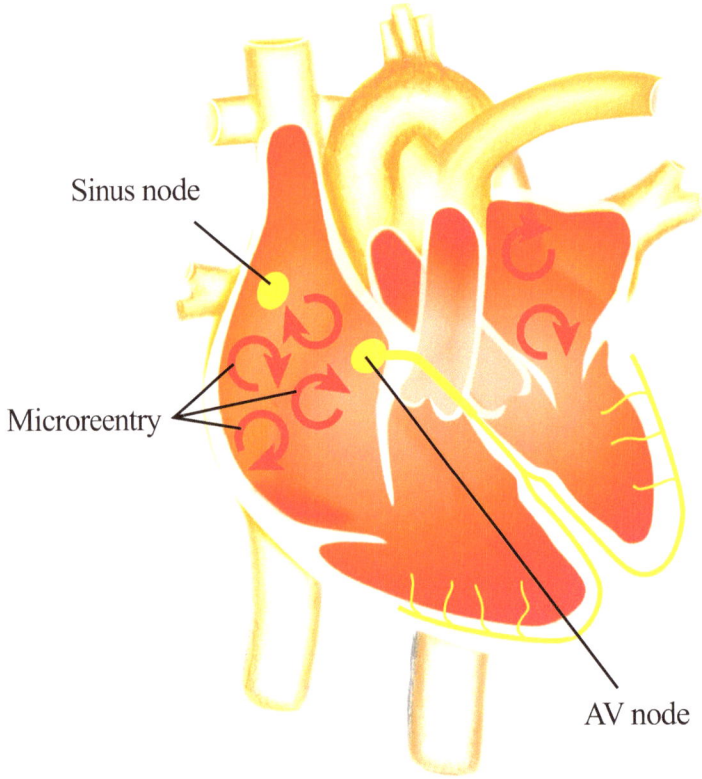

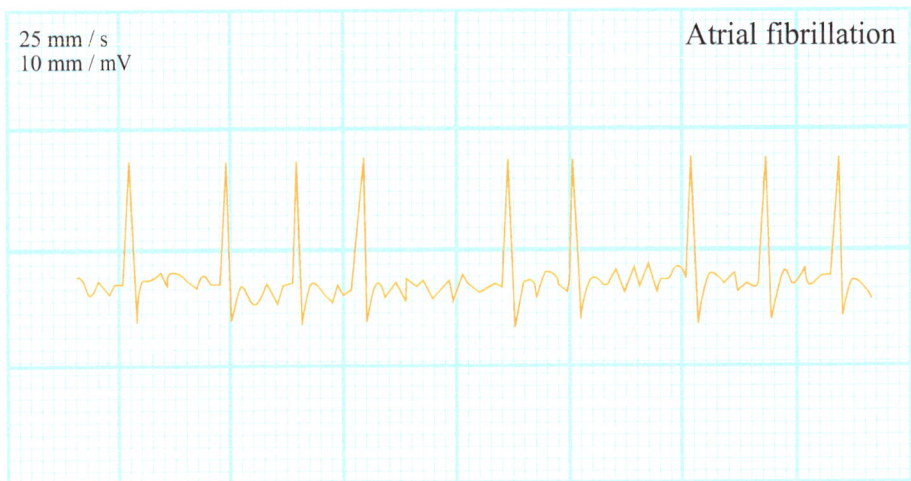

Figure 16: Irregularly irregular arrhythmia with oscillation of the baseline in AF.

QRS complexes are usually narrow unless conduction abnormalities like BBB are associated with AF. Intermittent BBB, mainly RBBB, can occur in AF and reflects some functional conduction disturbances known as Ashman phenomenon. Ashman beats are described as wide complex QRS complexes that follow a short R-R interval preceded by a long R-R interval. This wide QRS complex typically has RBBB morphology and represents an aberrantly conducted complex that originates above the A-V node, rather than a complex that originates in either the right or left ventricle. It occurs because the duration of the refractory period of the myocardium is proportional to the R-R interval of the preceding cycle. A short R-R interval is associated with a shorter duration of action potential and *vice versa*. A long R-R cycle will prolong the ensuing refractory period, and if a shorter cycle follows, the beat terminating the cycle is likely to be conducted aberrantly. Because the refractory period of the right bundle branch is longer than that of the left, the right bundle will still be in its refractory period when the supraventricular impulse reaches the His-Purkinje system resulting in a complex with right bundle branch morphology (Fig. **19**).

Tachy-Brady Syndrome

Periods of fast arrhythmias (supraventricular tachycardias), especially atrial fibrillation or atrial flutter, alternating with periods of very slow heart rates constitute the typical findings of the tachy-brady syndrome. The diagnosis is ususally made on a 24 hours recording. Tachy-brady syndrome is part of the group of sick sinus syndrome arrhythmias [3, 5].

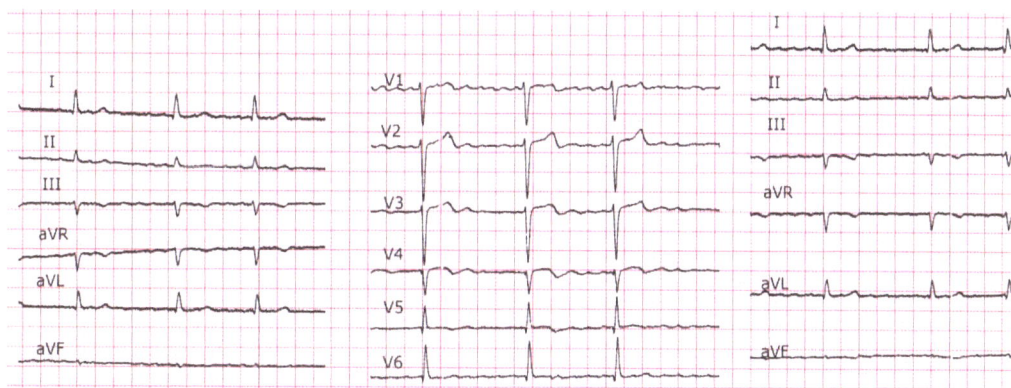

Figure 17: Atrial fibrillation with irregularly irregular rhythm. Mean ventricular rate at approximately 60 bpm.

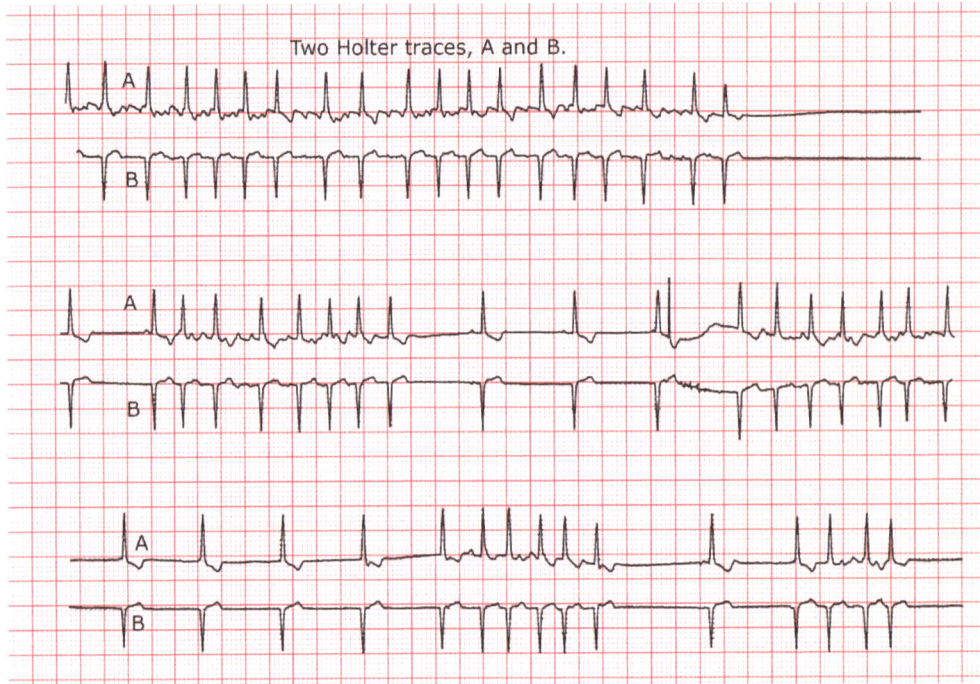

Figure 18: Holter monitoring wih alternating atrial tachycardia, atrial fibrillation and sinus rhythm. Some QRS complexes are not preceded by P waves corresponding to a nodal escape rhythm. This arrhythmia, occuring without underlying heart disease, is called focal atrial fibrillation. It is due to focal ectopic activity arising from the junction of the pulmonary veins and the left atrium. The first choice treatment of this arrhythmia is radiofrequency catheter ablation.

AV Nodal Tachycardia (Junctional)

AV nodal reentrant tachycardia (AVNRT) is also called junctional tachycardia. AVNRT is usually a reentrant tachycardia using a reentry circuit located within the AV node area. Rarely, the mechanism is an automatic tachycardia originating in the A-V junction. It tends to be a regular, narrow complex tachycardia and may be a sign of digitalis toxicity.

In the typical form of AVNRT (> 90% of the cases), the reentry circuit uses the slow pathway antegradely and the fast pathway retrogradely [6]. Antegrade ventricular activation occurs simultaneously with the retrograde atrial activation. The P' wave is hidden in the QRS complex, sometimes visible as a small r' wave in V1 at the end of the QRS complex. Rarely it can be seen as a small q wave in the inferior leads (Fig. **20**) Comparison of the trace in tachycardia and in sinus rhythm facilitates the diagnosis unless conduction abnormalities (BBB) are present during tachycardia.

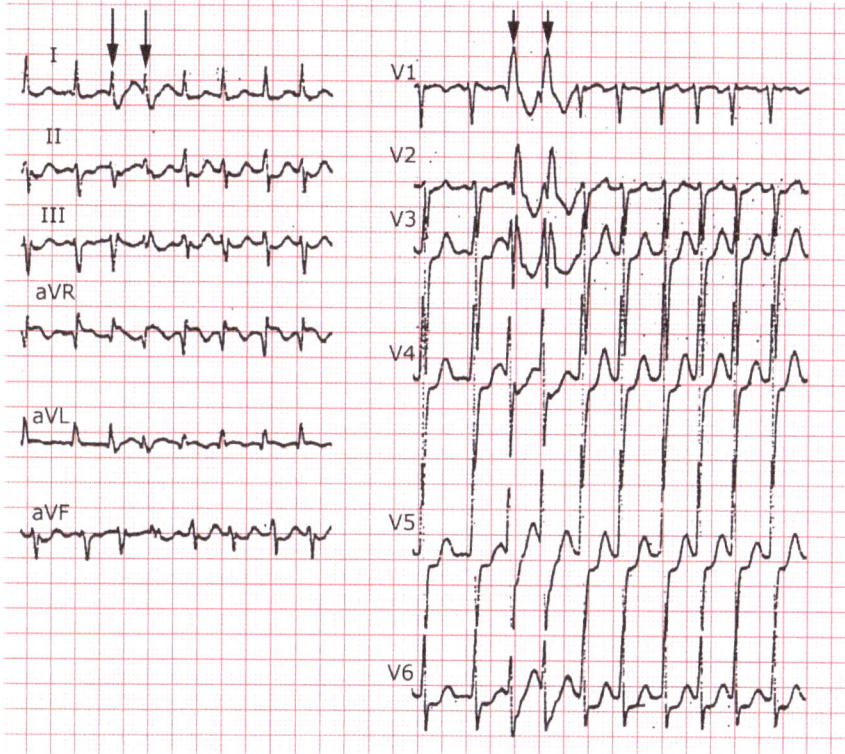

Figure 19: Atrial fibrillation with 2 consecutive (arrows) wide QRS complexes (RBBB) typical of the Ashman phenomenon.

In the atypical form (5-10%of cases), the reentry circuit uses the fast pathway antegradely and the slow pathway retrogradely. The P' wave is negative in the inferior leads with a ratio P'R/ RP'< 1 as in atrial tachycardia from which it should be differentiated.

It is rare for a nodal tachycardia to be automatic but when this is the case it is not completely regular. P' waves are either invisible or hidden within the terminal portion of the QRS complexes as with reentry.

The rate of typical AVNRT is between 160 and 220 bpm. AV condution is usually 1:1 but when the tachycardia initiates a 2:1 functional block can be seen. The trace is pathognomonic with negative P' waves in the inferior limb leads located exactly in the middle of the RR inteval. The RR interval is between 80 and 110 bpm (Fig. **21**). A-V 1:1 conduction occurs after a few seconds, often with functional aberrant conduction of the RBBB type (Fig. **22**).

Finally the negative P' wave is situated exactly in the middle of the RR interval when conduction is slow in both antegrade and retrograde pathways. This tachycardia is called "slow-slow".

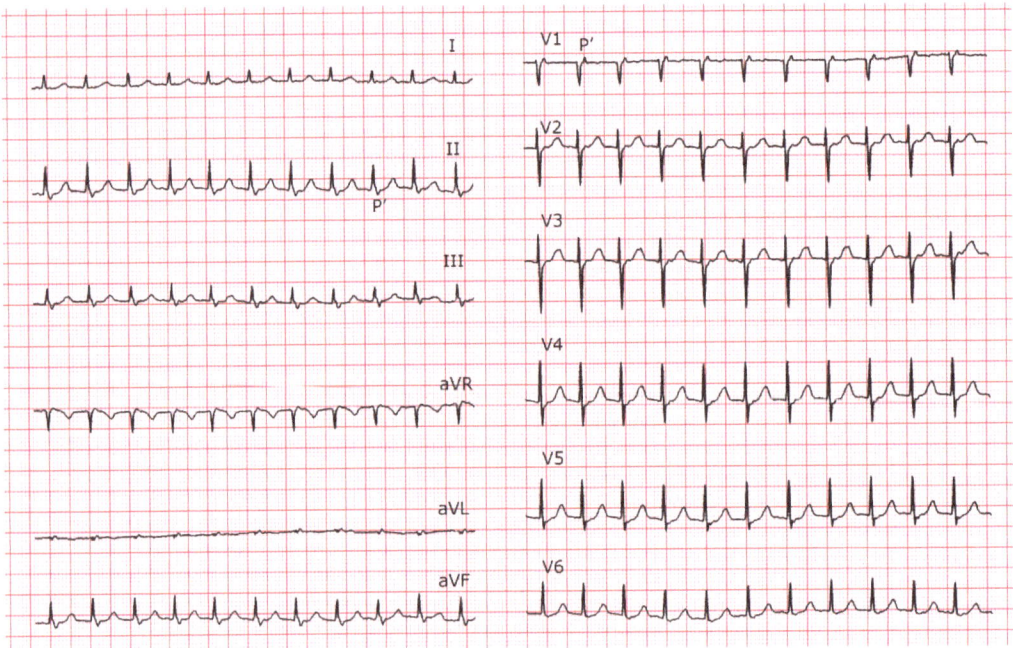

Figure 20: Typical AV nodal tachycardia at 150 bpm. At the end of the QRS complex a P' wave is visible, negative in II, III and aVF, because of retrograde activation of the atrium. In V1 this small P' wave is the r wave at the end of the QRS complex.

Atrioventricular Reentrant Tachycardia

Wolff-Parkinson-White Syndrome (WPW)

In the normal heart, electrical signals use only one pathway to propagate through the heart. This is the atrio-ventricular or A-V node. If there is an extra conduction pathway present, the electrical signal may arrive at the ventricle too soon. This condition is called Wolff-Parkinson-White syndrome (WPW). It is in a category of electrical abnormalities called "pre-excitation syndromes" (Fig. **23**). The electrical properties of this pathway, which is basically an abnormal muscular connection between the atrium and the ventricle, are different from those of the normal A-V conduction system and creates the conditions for a reentry circuit. The accessory pathway can conduct exclusively antegradely, in other words from the atrium to the ventricle, exclusively retrogradely, from the ventricle to the atrium or in a bidirectional manner. It can be located anywhere in the A-V groove but predominantely in the lateral region.

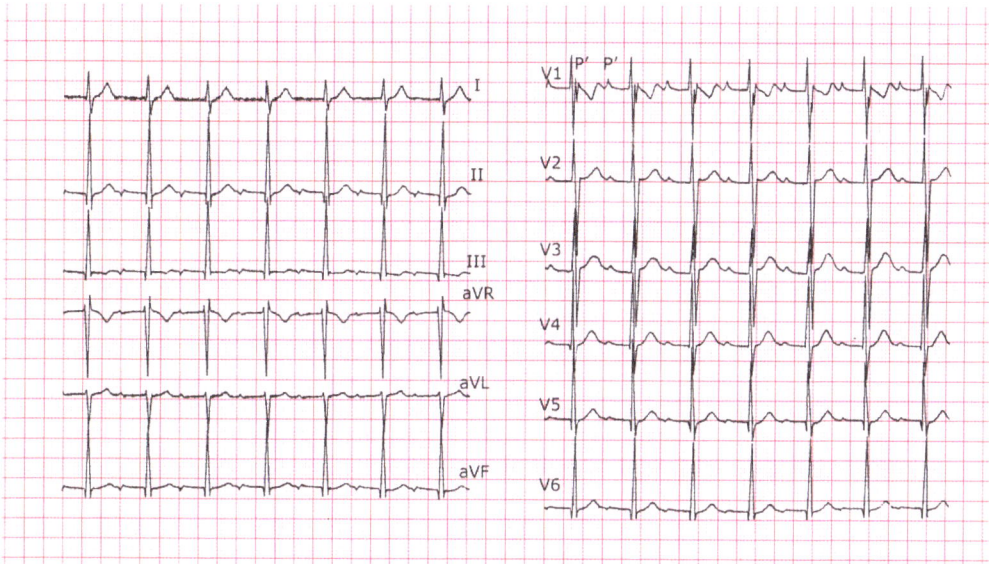

Figure 21: AV nodal tachycardia with 2:1 A-V block. In the middle of the RR interval a P' wave is seen. At the end of the QRS complex a small terminal r wave is seen in V1 and also represents a P' wave.

Sinus Rhythm

In individuals with antegrade conduction over the accessory pathway, electrical activity that is initiated in the sinus node travels through the accessory pathway as well as through the A-V node to activate the ventricles *via* both pathways. Since the accessory pathway does not have the impulse-slowing properties of the A-V node, the electrical impulse first activates the ventricles *via* the accessory pathway, and immediately afterwards *via* the A-V node. This gives the short PR interval and slurred upstroke to the QRS complex known as the delta wave or preexcitation. The PR interval is short (< 120 ms), the QRS complex is prolonged (> 120 ms) and the repolarisation is abnormal (Fig. **23**). The QRS duration, morphology and prominence of the ∂ wave are related to the participation of the accessory pathway to the ventricular activation. When most of this activation results from the normal A-V pathways the QRS complex is almost normal. When antegrade conduction is temporarily or permanently absent the accessory pathway is termed a "concealed acceossory pathway". The ∂ wave is absent and ventricular activation occurs *via* the normal A-V pathway.

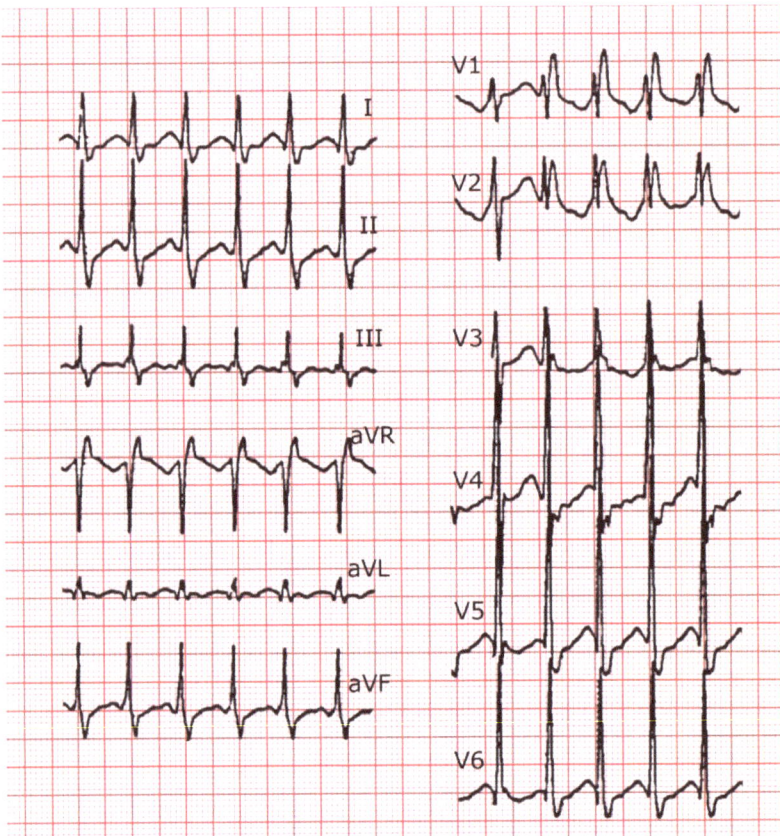

Figure 22: AV nodal tachycardia with functional RBBB. The first beat (on the left) in V1 is normal without QRS prolongation. The frequency of the tachycardia is the same with narrow and prolonged QRS complex duration. This is an argument favouring nodal tachycardia witth aberrant conduction.

The majority of accessory pathways are left sided. Patients with WPW often exhibit more than one accessory pathway, as is seen in patients with cardiac malformations such as for example Ebstein's anomaly. Other accessory pathways have been described, such as nodo-ventricular pathways. They are rarely seen clinically and diagnosis usually requires further electrophysiological testing.

Accessory pathways with antegrade conduction often exhibit retrograde conduction. In some patients, multiple accessory pathways can be present; the QRS complex will exhibit several morphologies depending on the participation of each accessory pathway in the preexcitation of the ventricles. This depends on the localization of the accessory pathways as well as on their refractory periods and on the autonomic tone. Tachycardias provoked by multiple accessory pathways pose a challenge in the interpretation of the trace.

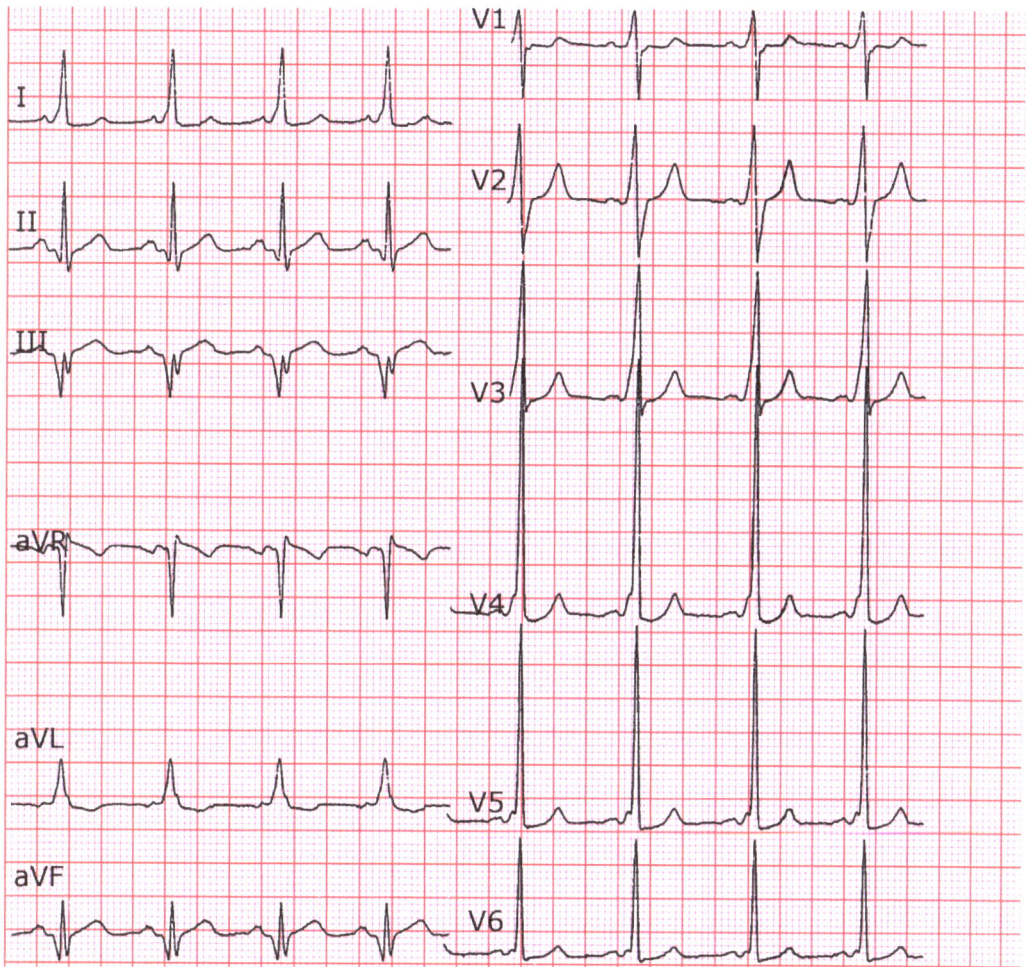

Figure 23: WPW syndrome in sinus rhythm (left postero-septal accessory pathway based on the morphology of the ∂ wave (see Table **1**). A short PR or PQ interval with a ∂ wave can be seen. In the presence of preexcitation, changes in the terminal portion of the QRS have no diagnostic value: they are simply the result of abnormal depolarisation. It is important to avoid the pitfall of interpreting these changes as ischemia. The Q waves do not indicate myocardial necrosis.

Tachycardia

Orthodromic Tachycardia

Orthodromic tachycardia is the most common arrhythmia associated with accessory pathways. It is a macro-reentry circuit using the A-V node antegradely and the accesory pathway retrogradely. Passage through this accessory pathway delays the retrograde activation of the atrium. This manifests, on the ECG, as a time delay between the QRS complex and the next P' wave (> 100 ms) (Fig. **24**).

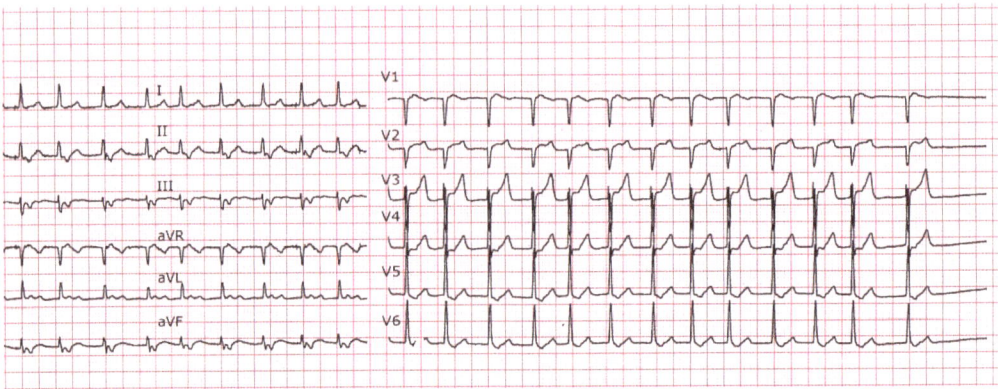

Figure 24: Orthodromic tachycardia with narrow QRS complex and a P' wave distant from the QRS complex (120 ms) and negative in II, III and aVF with a ratio RP'/P'R< 1. The acccessory pathway is located in the inferior A-V groove.

The position of the P' wave is the main difference between AVNRT and orthodromic tachycardia using an accessory pathway. In the latter, the P' wave is visible between the QRS complexes and in AV nodal reentrant tachycardia the P' wave is hidden in the QRS complex. In orthodromic tachycardia the RP' interval represents retrograde conduction through the accessory pathway (fast conduction) and the P'R interval denotes antegrade conduction through the A-V node (slow conduction). Localization of the accessory pahtway is possible based on the axis of the P' wave: the accessory pathway is left lateral with a negative P' wave in I and aVL; it is inferior with a negative P' wave in II, III and aVF. QRS alternans is often seen in orthodromic tachycardia and is very suggestive of this arrhythmia (Fig. **25**). Only 10% of atrial tachycardias and 2% of AV nodal tachycardias exhibit QRS alternans. Conversely when QRS alternans is present the probability of an orthodromic tachycardia using an accesssory pathway is 90%.

QRS complexes can be narrow, or wide when aberrant conduction is present. It is usually a LBBB although in AV nodal reentrant tachycardia RBBB is more frequent (Fig. **26**). In wide QRS complex tachycardia the P' wave is most often invisible, because it is hidden in the QRS. An algorithm can help to differentiate ventricular tachycardia from wide QRS complex supraventricular tachycardia.

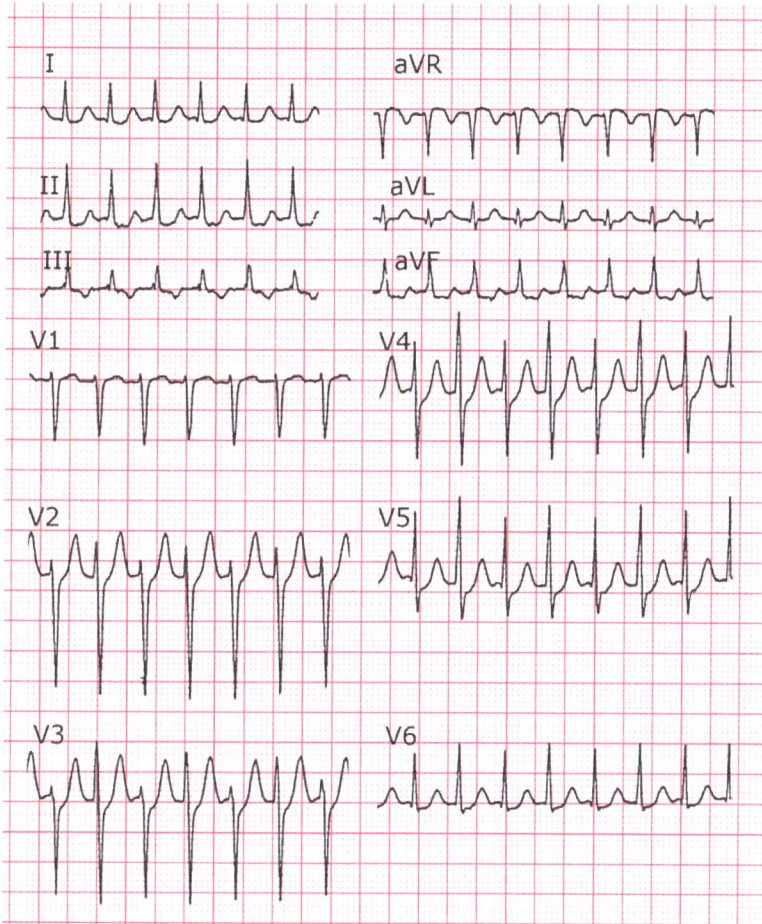

Figure 25: Narrow QRS complex tachycardia. QRS alternans is present in all leads. P' waves visible in II and III with a ratio RP'/P'R < 1.

Aberrant conduction during orthodromic tachycardia helps in the localization of the accessory pathway. An ipsilateral accessory pahtway prolongs the cycle length of the tachycardia (slower heart rate). For example if a LBBB prolongs the cycle length of the tachycardia, the accessory pathway is left sided. The block is called "slowing block". This is due to a prolongation of the reentry circuit induced by the block. The activation has to travel through the right branch of the His bundle and through the septum before reaching the accessory pathway. A RBBB will not change the cycle length of a tachycardia with a left sided accessory pathway.

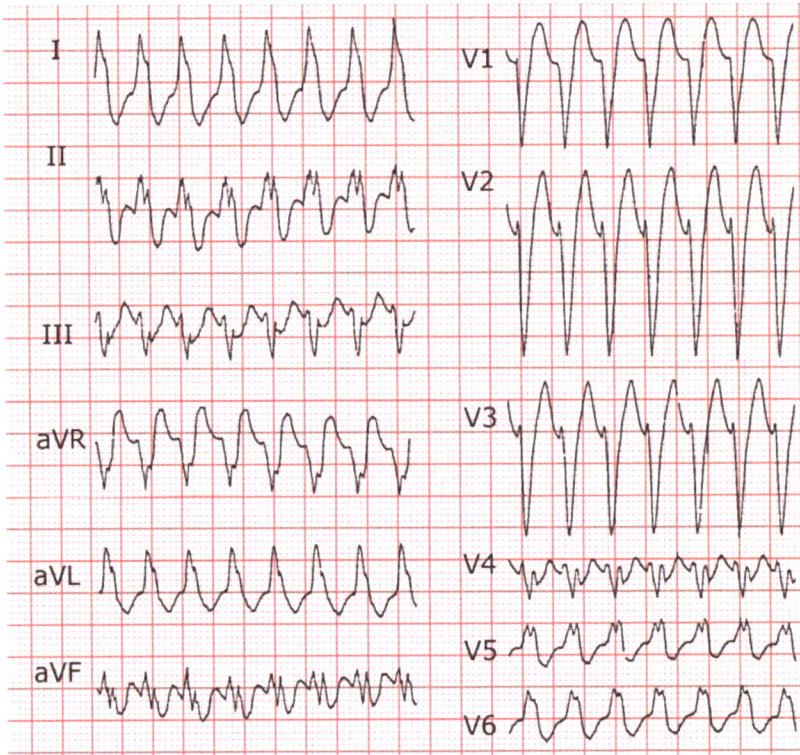

Figure 26: Orthodromic tachycardia using an acessory pathway with aberrant conduction of the type LBBB. As P' waves are not visible the algorithm used for differentiation of wide QRS tachycardias can be used to determine the mechanism of the tachycardia.

Antidromic Tachycardia

Less commonly, a shorter refractory period in the accessory tract may cause block of an ectopic atrial impulse in the normal A-V pathway, with antegrade conduction down the accessory tract and then retrograde conduction up the normal (A-V) pathway. This type of tachycardia produced is called antidromic tachycardia. The QRS complex is wide (> 140 ms), with an exaggeration of the delta wave seen during sinus rhythm (wide-QRS tachycardia) (Fig. **27**). Such tachycardias are difficult to differentiate from ventricular tachycardia.

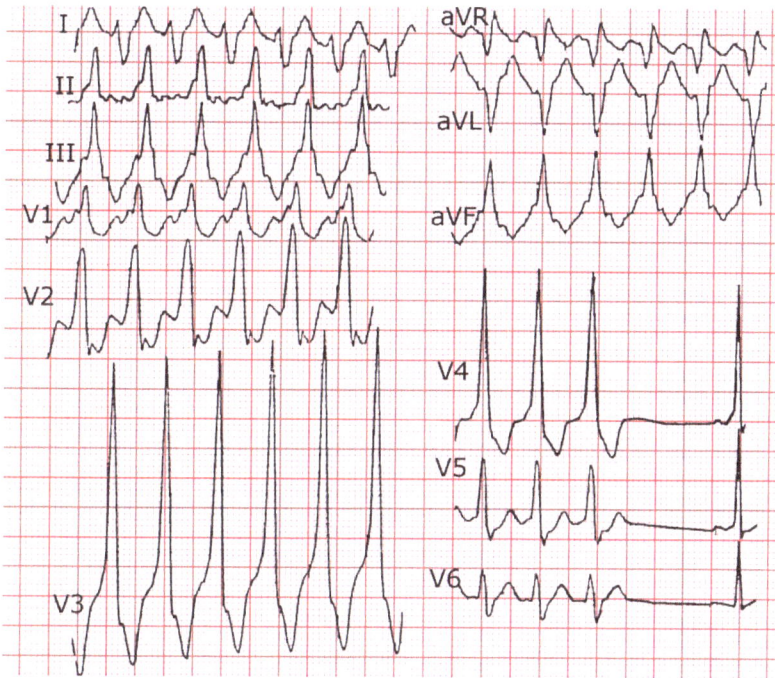

Figure 27: Antidromic tachycardia with wide QRS complexes (140 ms). Retrograde P' waves are hidden in the QRS complex. The following beat following tachycardia interruption (V4-V6) shows the typical patterns of the WPW syndrome with a short PR interval and a ∂ wave.

Atrial Fibrillation

Atrial fibrillation is the third arrhythmia occuring in patients with accessory pathways. The depolarisation can reach the ventricles by both the normal A-V pathway and the accessory pathway. If the latter has a short refractory period and as conduction can be very fast over this accessory pathway, the ventricular response can be very high, up to 300 bpm and irregular. The QRS complexes are wide but with a variable width depending on the use of the accessory pathway by the depolarisation. This is a dangerous arrhythmia since the high heart rate is hemodynamically poorly tolerated. Ventricular fibrillation may occur in young patients and lead to sudden death (Fig. **28**).

The ECG patterns of the ∂ wave allow localization of the accessory pathway on the surface ECG. Localization of the accessory pahtway using the QRS and , ∂ wave axis is possible provided the QRS complex duration is > 120 ms. Finally the axis of the ∂ wave must be concordant with the axis of the QRS complex and the difference between these 2 axes should not be over 30°otherwise the presence of 2 accessory pathways must be suspected. The following Table **1** gives some clues aiding accessory pathway localization.

Table 1: Location of the accessory pathway

Derivation	Left lateral	Postero-septal	Right lateral	Antero-septal
I	0, -	+	+	+
II	+	-,0	+	+
III	+	-	+,0,-	+
aVL	-	+	+	+
aVF	+	-	+	+
V1	+	+,0,_	-,0	-
V2	+	+	0,+	-
V6	-,0,+	+	+	+

Abbreviations: LG = left lateral location of the accessory pathway. PS = postero-septal location. LD = right lateral location. AS = antero-septal location. ∂ = wave negative.∂ = wave positive. 0 = ∂ wave isoelectric.

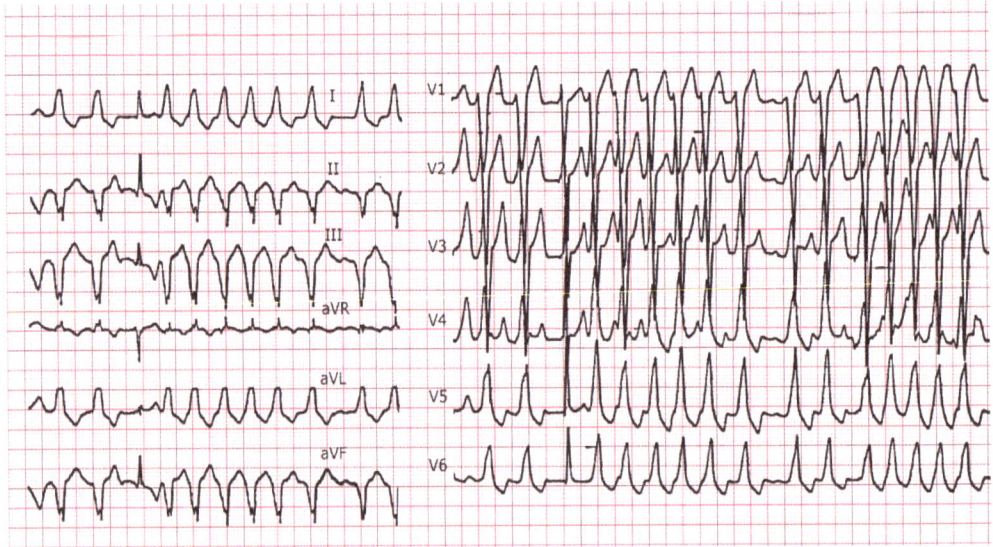

Figure 28: Atrial fibrillation in a patient with WPW syndrome. Variable width of the QRS comlex is present. The arrhythmia is irregularly irregular.

Summary of the arrhythmias associated with the WPW syndrome (Fig. **29**):

1. Sinus rhythm. The electrical activity that is initiated in the sinus node travels through the accessory pathway as well as through the A-V

node to activate the ventricles *via* both pathways. Since the accessory pathway does not have the impulse slowing properties of the A-V node, the electrical impulse first activates the ventricles *via* the accessory pathway, and immediately afterwards *via* the A-V node. This gives the short PR interval and the delta wave (fusion complex).

2. Orthodromic tachycardia. The electrical activity travels antegradely through the A-V node and retrogradely through the accessory pathway. QRS complexes are narrow unless a preexisitng or functional aberrant conduction is present.

3. Antidromic tahcycardia. Depolarisation uses the accessory pathway antegradely and the A-V node pathway retrogradely. The QRS complexes are wide.

4. Atrial fibrillation. QRS complexes are wide and irregularly irregular. QRS duration varies depending on the degree of fusion between the accessory pathway and the A-V node. If atrial fibrillation develops, the normal rate-limiting effects of the A-V node are bypassed, and the resultant excessive ventricular rates may lead to ventricular fibrillation. Impulses from the atria are conducted to the ventricles *via* either both of the A-V node and accessory pathway producing a broad fusion complex or just the AV node producing a narrow complex (without a delta wave) or just the accessory pathway producing a very broad 'pure' delta wave.

Permanent Junctional Reentrant Tachycardia (PJRT=Permanent Junctional Reentrant Tachycardia) (or Coumel Tachycardia)

Permanent junctional re-entrant tachycardia is a relatively uncommon form of re-entry tachycardia with antegrade conduction occurring through the atrioventricular node and retrograde conduction over an accessory pathway usually located in the postero-septal region. It is a macroreentry circuit using the A-V node antegradely and the accessory pathway retrogradely. The P'wave is negative in the limb leads with RP'>P'R (Fig. **30**). The heart rtate is not very high, usually between 100 and 150 bpm. Differential diagnosis includes low right atrial tachycardia and the atypical form of AV nodal reentrant tachycardia; all having RP'>P'R.

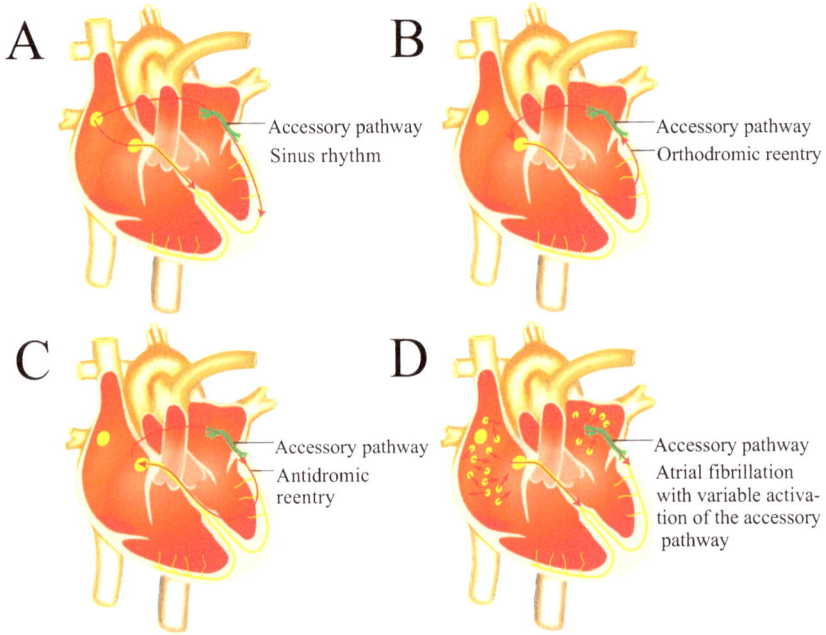

Figure 29: Arrhythmias associated with WPW syndrome.

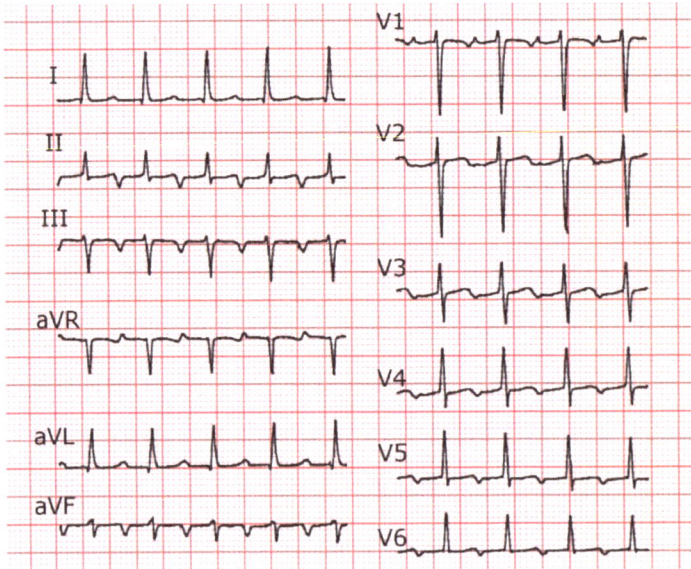

Figure 30: Classical PJRT with RP'/P'R > 1 and negative P' wave in II, III, aVF and from V3 to V6.

Narrow QRS Tachycardia Diagnostic Algorithm

Differentiation between several types of narrow QRS tachycardia, like atrial flutter, sinus tachycardia, AV nodal reentrant tachycardia or orthodromic tachycardia using an accessory pathway [1-3, 5, 7, 9] (Fig. **32**).

The following patterns have to be considered: heart rate, regularity or irregularity, morphology, polarity and position of the P wave (RP'/P'R), presence or otherwise of QRS alternans, A-V block provoked by vagal maneuvers. Finally, occurence of bundle branch block during the tachycardia may help to clinch the diagnosis.

Procedure to Determine the Mechanism of Narrow QRS Complex Tachycardias

1. Carotid sinus massage is useful for differentiating supraventricular tachycardias. Sudden interruption of the tachycardia is seen in: 1) orthodromic tachycardia 2) AV nodal reentrant tachycardia or rarely atrial tachycardia. When A-V block does not interrupt the tachycarida the underlying atrial activity emerges. Interruption of a permanent junctional reentrant tachycardia (PJRT) by carotid sinus massage is shown in Fig. **31**.

2. QRS alternans has been suggested as a marker of orthodromic tachycardia using an accessory pathway.

RP'/P'R Ratio (See Table 2)

1. <1: orthodromic tachycardia using a rapidly conducting accessory pathway or atrial tachycardia with slow A-V conduction.

2. =1: atrial tachycardia, typical AV nodal reentrant tachycardia with 2:1 block(the ventricular rate is between 90 and 110/min), AV nodal reentrant tachycardia "slow-slow".

3. >1: atypical nodal tachycardia, atrial tachycardia, orthodromic tachycardia using a slow conducting accessory pathway (PJRT).

4. No visible P' wave: typical AV nodal reentrant tachycardia. (See Fig. **31**).

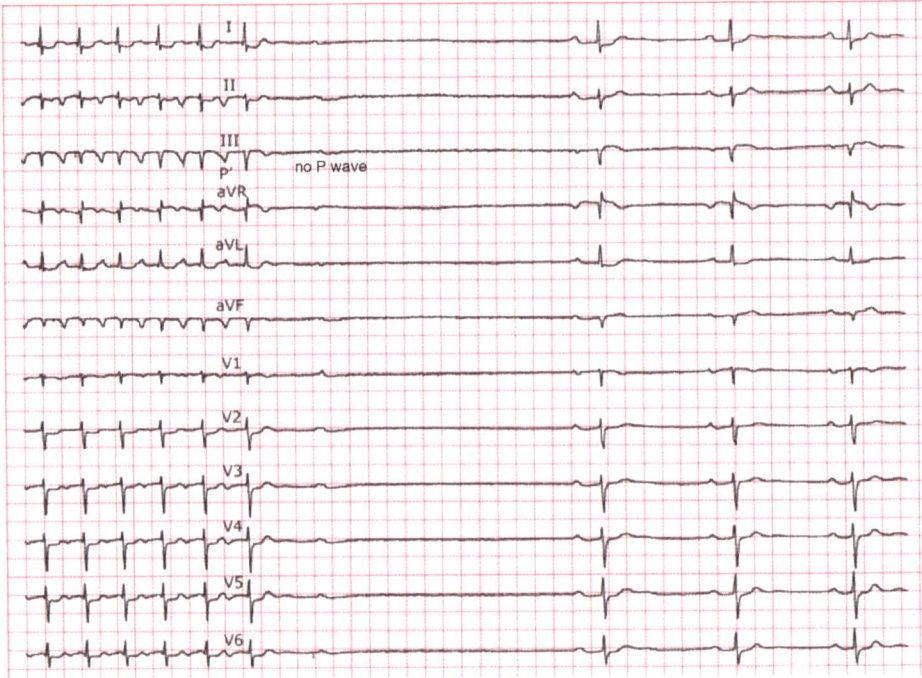

Figure 31: Permanent junctional reentrant tachycardia. A retrograde block (absence of P wave) is induced by carotid sinus massage followed by sinus rhythm and first degree A-V block.

P' Wave Morphology (see Table 2)

1. Negative in II, III, aVF: low right atrial tachycardia, atypical AV nodal reentrant tachycardia, orthodromic tachycardia over a postero-septal accessory pathway (see Table **2**).

2. Negative in I, aVL: orthodromic tachycardia over a left-sided accessory pathway, left atrial tachycardia.

3. Positive in II, III, aVF: atrial tachycardia.

Table 2: Narrow QRS complex tachycardia: differential diagnosis

ECG	Nodal	Orthodromic	Atrial	PJRT
AV block	(+)	-	++	-
Alternance	(+)	(+++)	(+)	-
P wave	Within QRS	RP'<P'R	Between QRS	RP'>P'R
P wave polarity	- in II, III, aVF	Variable	Variable	- in II,III, aVF
Aberrant conduction	+ (RBBB)	++ (LBBB)	+	-

a).

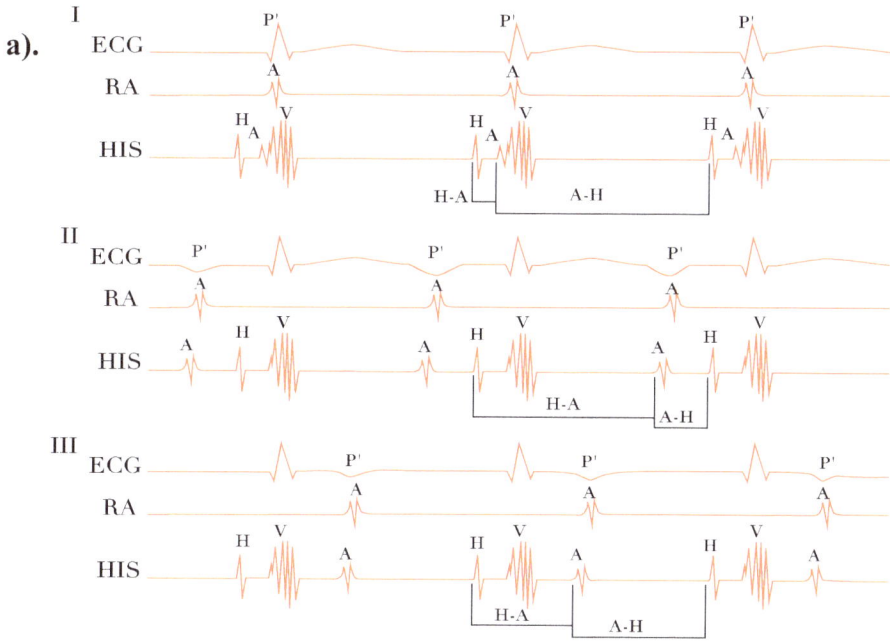

b). **Narrow QRS complex tachycardia: diagnostic algorithm**

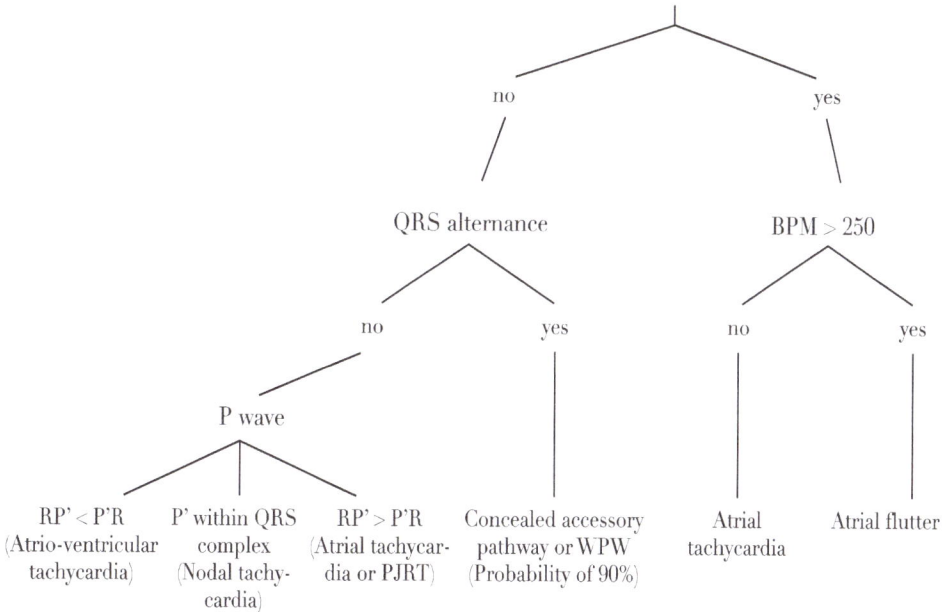

Figure 32: Localization of the P' wave in supraventricular tachycardia: (Endocardial recording, V = Ventriculogram A = Auriculogram). I: AV nodal reentrant tachycardia, II: atrial tachycardia or PJRT and III: atrioventricular reentrant tachycardia.

VENTRICULAR TACHYCARDIA

Three or more beats that originate from the ventricle at a rate of more than 100 beats per minute constitute a ventricular tachycardia. If the fast rhythm self-terminates within 30 seconds, it is considered a non-sustained ventricular tachycardia. If the rhythm lasts more than 30 seconds it is known as a sustained ventricular tachycardia (even if it terminates on its own after 30 seconds). Ventricular tachycardia can be classified based on its morphology: monomorphic ventricular tachycardia means that the appearance of all the beats matches each other in each lead of a surface electrocardiogram. Polymorphic ventricular tachycardia, on the other hand, has beat-to-beat variation in morphology. The most common cause of monomorphic ventricular tachycardia is damaged or dead (scar) tissue from a previous myocardial infarction. This scar cannot conduct electrical activity, so there is a potential circuit around the scar that results in the tachycardia. This is typically a re-entrant circuit like in atrial flutter and the re-entrant forms of supraventricular tachycardia. Other rare congenital causes of monomorphic VT include right ventricular dysplasia, and right and left ventricular outflow tract tachycardia. Less commonly, ventricular tachycardia occurs in individuals with structurally normal hearts. This is known as idiopathic ventricular tachycardia and confers little or no incidence of increased risk of sudden cardiac death. Idiopathic ventricular tachycardia ("idiopathic VT") is generally the type of VT seen in younger individuals diagnosed with VT. While the causes of idiopathic VT are not known, it is generally presumed to be congenital, and can be brought on by any number of diverse factors. The QRS complex is > 120 ms in more than 90% of ventricular tachycardia; rarely it can be < 120 ms in fascicular tachyardia. Localization of the site of origin of ventricular tahcycardia can be determined with the QRS morphology during tachycardia.

A-V Dissociation

Atrial activity is generally under the control of the sinus node during venricular tachycardia but is completely independent of the ventricular activity. This is called A-V dissociation and is characterised by different PP and RR intervals (Fig. **33**).

1. ***Retrograde conduction***: in 20% of cases, retrograde (ventriculo-atrial) conduction is present: negative P' waves in the limb leads can be

identified sometimes with retrograde Wenckebach conduction or even a 2:1 retrograde block.

2. ***Antegrade conduction***: is intermittent represented by fusion and capture beats. They are excellent criteria for the diagnosis of ventricular tachycardia. Rarely atrial arrhythmias are present with ventricular tachycardia (atrial fibrillation, flutter or tachycardia) and are termed "bi-tachycardia". Atrial activity can be hidden by the ventricular activity (broad QRS complexes) (Fig. **34**). This emphasizes the value of A-V dissociation in the diagnosis of ventricular tachycardia.

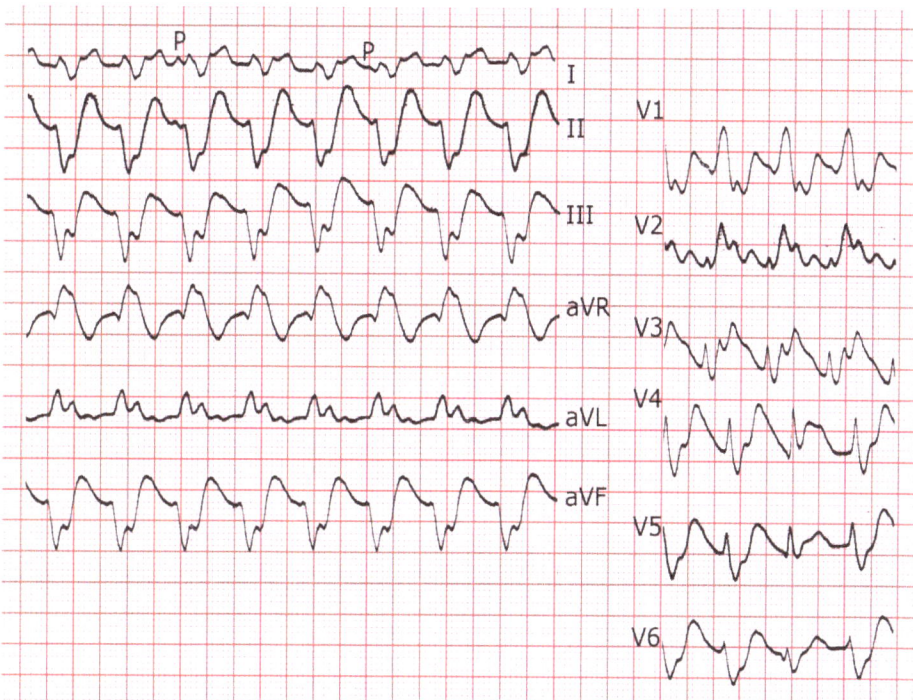

Figure 33: Ventricular tachycardia. A-V dissociation and typical appearance of the QRS complex is present.

3. ***Capture***: an atrial activity reaching the ventricles out of their refractory period is transmitted normally to the ventricles. The QRS complex is narrow and is intercalated between broad QRS complexes and is called a capture beat (Fig. **34**).

4. ***Fusion***: as for capture beat the atrial activity is transmitted to the ventricles partially depolarized through the A-V node. The resulting complex shape is between a narrow and a broad QRS complex called a fusion beat (Figs. **35** and **36**).

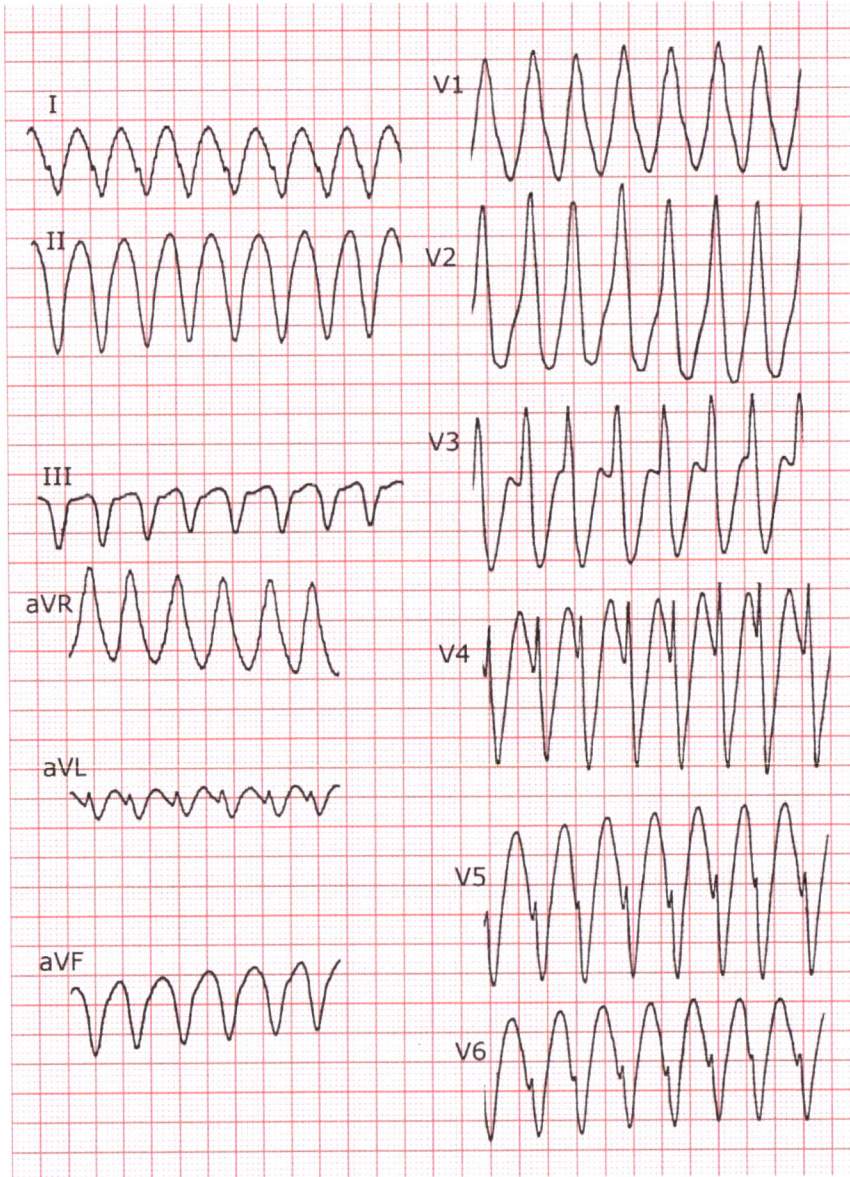

Figure 34: Ventricular tachycardia without visible P waves. Only the morphology of the QRS complex can be used in the diagnosis.

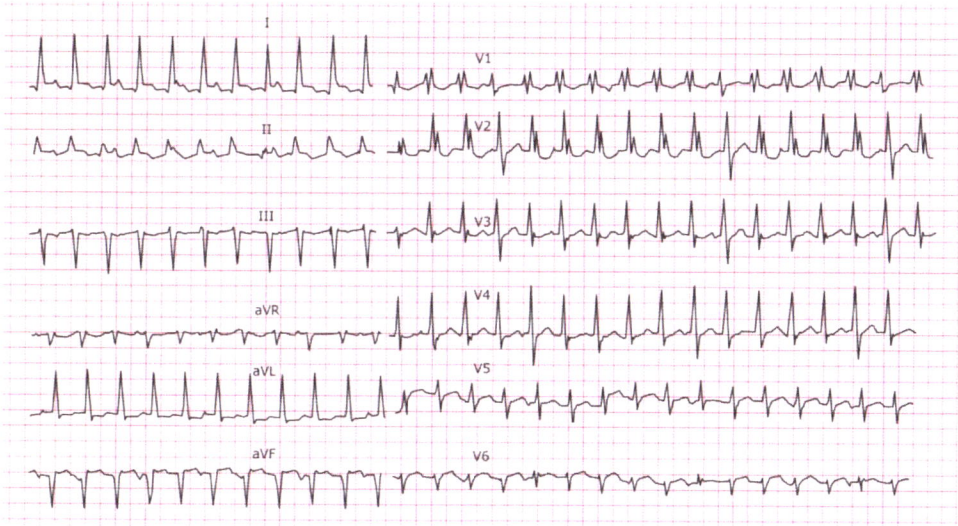

Figure 35: Wide QRS complex with A-V disociation and fusion beats during venrticular tachycardia. The QRS complexes are not very broad because the tachycardia arises from the upper septum close to the normal A-V conduction system.

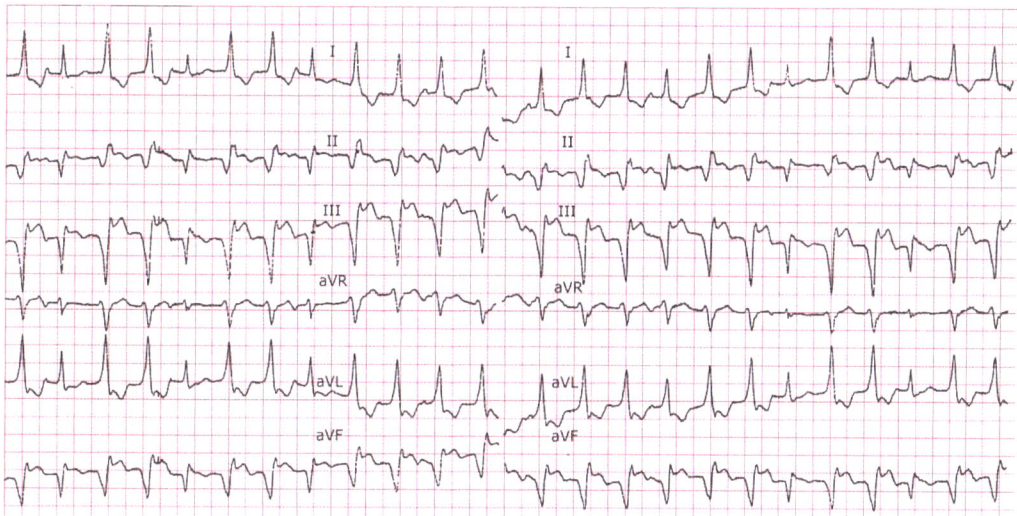

Figure 36: A-V dissociation with fusion and capture beats typical of ventricular tachycardia.

Distinction between ventricular tachycardia from antidromic tachycardia may be difficult. In both situations ventricular activation occurs outside of the normal A-V conduction system, directly from the myocardium. However, a predominant S wave from V4 to V6 or a qR morphology from V2 to V6 favors the diagnosis of ventricular tachycardia.

Idiopathic Ventricular Tachycardia

Idiopathic ventricular tachycardias include tachycardias arising from the right or left infudibulum ("outflow tract") and fasicular tachycardias.

Right or left outflow tract tachycardia (RVOT) has a LBBB morphology (predominant S wave in V1) with a vertical QRS complex axis although left outflow tract tachycardia (sometimes arising from the Valsalva sinus) has RBBB morphology, (predominant R wave in V1) and a vertical QRS complex axis (Fig. **37**). Left outflow tract tachycardia (LVOT) has also been described. Differential diagnosis between these 2 types of tachycardia is based on the morphology of the QRS complex in V2. V2 transition ratios ≥ 0.60 predict an LVOT origin (V2 ratio = percentage R-wave during VT (R/R+S) VT divided by the percentage R-wave in sinus rhythm (R/R+S)). In addition a premature ventricular contraction precordial transition occurring later than the sinus rhythm transition excludes an LVOT origin with 100% accuracy.

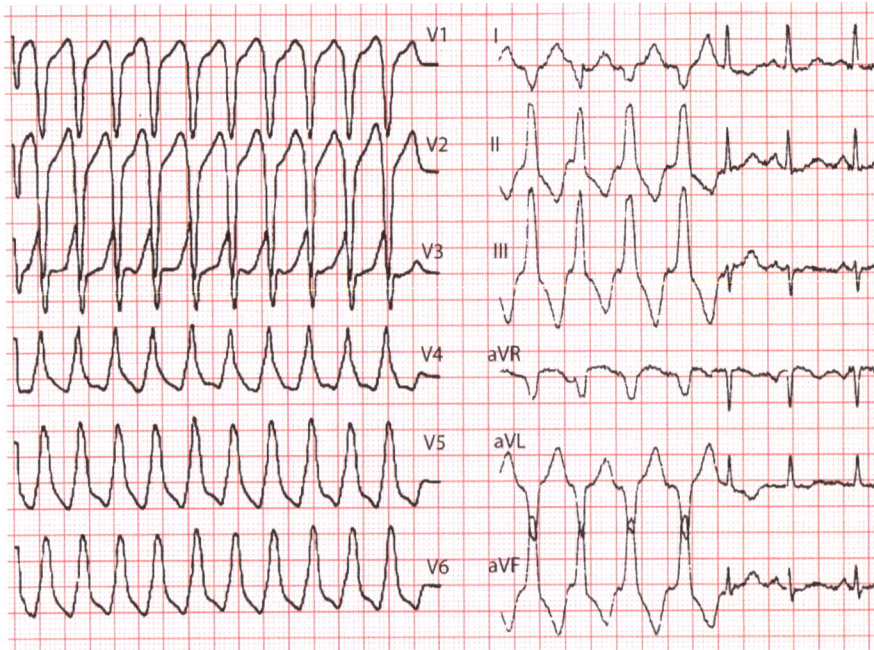

Figure 37: Ventricular tachycardia arising from the right outflow tract. The precordial leads are on the left. The aspect of the QRS complex in the limb leads in typical of an outflow tract tachycardia. The aspect of the QRS complex in V2 is compatible with a right side origin. VT spontaneously stopped during the recording as shown on the right part of the trace.

Fascicular tachycardias arise from the conduction fibres of the heart. Tachycardias arising from the left posterior fascicle have RBBB morphology with left axis deviation and RBBB morphology with right axis deviation when arising from the left anterior fascicle. These tachycardias have a good prognosis. However, R on T phenomenom degenerating into ventricular fibrillation, causing sudden death, has been occasionally described.

Arrhyhthmogenic Right Ventricuar Dysplasia

This is a rare disease of the young adult. Fibro-fatty tissue replaces the normal myocardium and causes electrical inhomogeneity and instability. This favors reentry mechanism and tachycardias. These tachycardias have LBBB morphology with variable axis. Sudden death is the major risk associated with this disease. T waves are inverted in V2, V3 and a small notch at the end of the S wave can be seen in V1-V2 (€ wave). Ventricular premature contractions with a LBBB morphology are also typically associatedwith this disease (Fig. **38**).

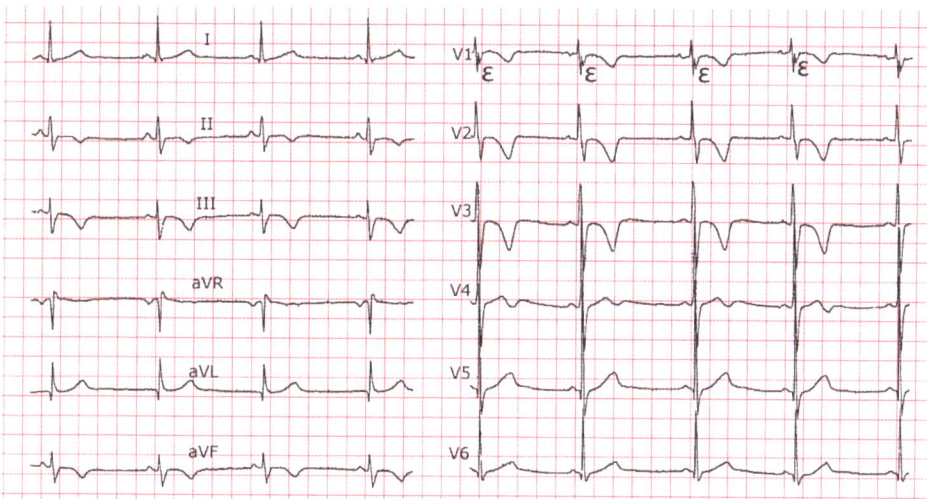

Figure 38: Right ventricular dysplasia with € wave in V1 and negative T waves from V1 to V3 can be seen.

Differential Diagnosis of Wide QRS Complexes Tachycardias

The electrical activity in ventricular tachycardia, unlike in supraventricular tachycardia with aberrant conduction, arises from the ventricular muscle and not from the His-Purkinje system. Thus the QRS complex is significantly wider than the QRS complex of aberrant conduction because of the difference in conduction velocity between the His-Purkinje system and the ventricular muscle His-Purkinje. This difference in the excitation patterns is mainly seen at the beginnning of the QRS complex. As a result, most of the criteria used for the diagnosis of ventricular tahcycardia are based upon the initial QRS complex morphology: rapid deflection and sudden upstroke in abberant condution or slow deflection in ventricular tachycardia.

Wide QRS complex tachycardias include ventricular tachycardias, orthodromic tachycardias with aberrant conduction and antidromic tachycardias. Ventricular tachycardias are the most frequent (80%), followed by tachycardias with aberrant conduction (15-20%) and finally rarely antidromic tachycardias. Several algorithms have been proposed to differentiate these tachycardias. None of them is 100% reliable. They use some aspects of the complex like morphology, axis and duration and the atrial activity (Fig. **39**) [1-3, 5, 7, 9, 10].

Key Points (Fig. 39)

1. The rate of the tachycardia is not a criterion to differentiate ventricular tachycardia from supraventricular tachycardia. Ventricular tachycardia is usually regular except at the beginning when it can be irregular. Atrial flutter with 2:1 A-V conduction should always come to mind with a tachycardia of 150 bpm irrespective of the QRS duration.

2. QRS complex morphology in V1: a predominant S wave is called"left bundle type" whilst a predominant R wave is called "right bundle type". A QS appearance in all precordial leads is termed negative concordance and a monophasic R wave in all the precordial leads is termed positive concordance.

3. Wide QRS complex tachycardias not fullfilling the criteria for bundle branch block or fascicular block must be considered as ventricular tachycardia.

4. A 12 lead ECG must be recorded during tachycardia unless hemodynamic instability necessitates urgent cardioversion. In patients with ischemic heart disease, wide QRS complex tachycardia has a

ventricular origin in more than 95% of cases. Good hemodynamic tolerance can be seen in both supraventricular and ventricular tachycardias; this does not represent a criterion of discrimination.

QRS Aspect During Supraventricular Tachycardia and Aberrant Conduction

Right bundle branch block (RBBB)

- QRS triphasic in V1 and V6

- rSR appearance in V1 and qRs in V6.

- R/S >1 in V6.

Left bundle branch block (LBBB)

- r wave < 30 ms in V1 and V2.

- Rapid descent without notching of the S wave in V1 and V2.

- < 60 ms between the beginning of the QRS complex and the nadir of the S wave in V1 and V2.

Elements Suggesting Ventricular Tachycardia

QRS axis

- Axis between -90° and -180°(extreme right axis deviation).

- Axis < -30° with RBBB morphology.

- Axis > 90° with LBBB morphology.

QRS duration

- QRS > 140ms with RBBB morphology.

- QRS > 160ms with LBBB morphology.

- QRS in tachycardia > QRS in sinus rhythm.

QRS aspect

- QRS aspect not compatible with RBBB, LBBB or fascicular block morphology.

- Negative concordance from V1 to V6.

- Positive concordance from V1 to V6.

- Bundle branch block QRS morphology in tachycardia different from the BBB morphology in sinus rhythm.

Other criteria of ventricular tachycardia

- Without positive or negative concordance: interval between the beginnning of the r wave and the nadir of the S wave > 100 ms in one precordial lead.

- Initial R wave in aVR.

- R wave peak time $\geq$ 50 milliseconds in II.

- QR morphology (except in aVR).

- RBBB morphology:

In V1: - monophasic complex or qR morphology or triphasic complex with r' < R

In V6: - r/S < 1.

- LBBB morphology:

In V1 or V2: - r wave > 40

- Notch in the descending part of the S wave.

- Duration > 60 ms from the beginning of the QRS complex to the nadir of the S wave.

In V6: - Any q wave or QS

- The ratio between the initial activation speed and the terminal activation speed of the QRS complex ≤1; values are expressed in mV during the initial 40 ms and the 40 ms of the terminal portion of a bi- or multiphasic QRS complex with an abrupt upstroke and the most rapid initial activation (usually measured in the precordial leads).

- In lead aVR the following criteria can be used to confirm the ventricular origin of the tachycardia:

1. Presence of an initial R wave,

2. Width of an initial r or q wave > 40 ms,

3. Notching on the initial downstroke of a predominantly negative QRS complex,

4. Ventricular activation–velocity ratio (vi/vt) the vertical excursion (in millivolts) recorded during the initial (vi) and terminal (vt) 40 ms of the QRS complex.

- When any of criteria 1 to 3 is present, ventricular tachycardia is diagnosed; when absent, the next criterion is analyzed. In step 4, vi/vt > 1 suggests supraventricular tachycardia, and vi/vt < 1 suggests ventricular tachycardia.

Ventricular Flutter

QRS complexes and T waves are submerged into a regular sinusoidal wave in all leads, with a frequency between 250 and 300 beats per minute (Fig. **40**).

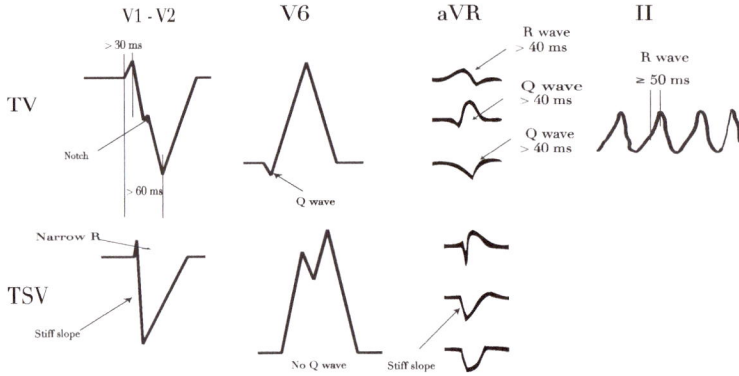

Figure 39: Morphologies of the QRS complex in V1, V2, V6 and aVR allowing differentiation of ventricular tachycardia (VT) from supraventricular tachycardia (SVT).

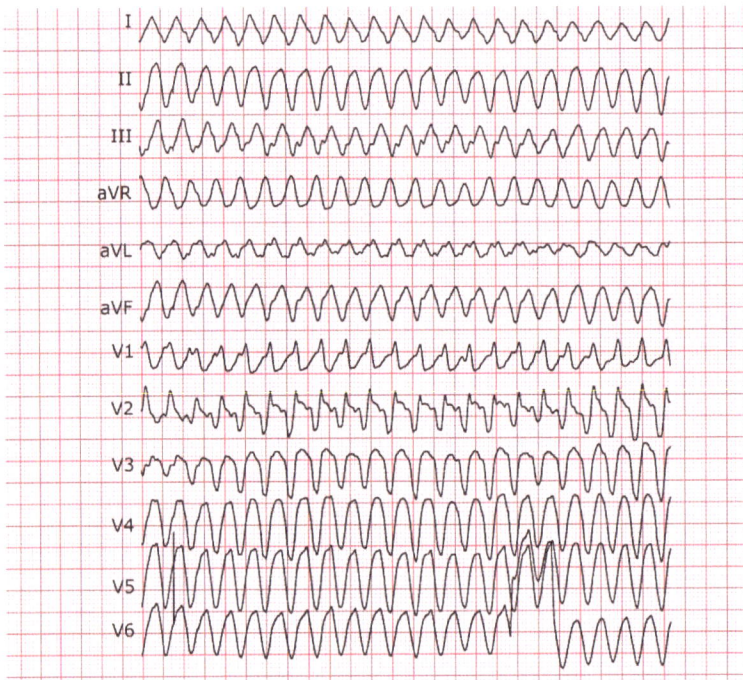

Figure 40: Ventricular flutter.

Accelerated Idioventricular Rhythm (A.I.V.R.)

AIVR often occurs during the acute phase of myocardial infarction and is a sign of reperfusion. It appears similar to ventricular tachycardia but is benign and does not need any treatment. It can most easily be distinguished from VT in that the rate is less than 120 and usually less than 100 bpm. Capture beats and fusion are frequent [1, 3, 7, 9] (Fig. **41**).

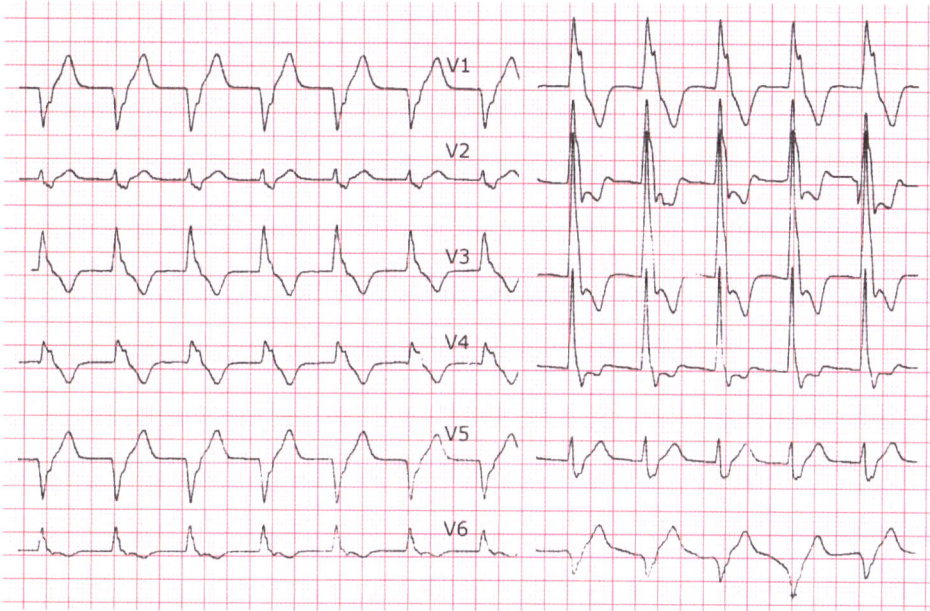

Figure 41: Accelerated idioventricular rhythm (AIVR).

Torsades de Pointes

Torsades de pointes or torsades, literally means "twisting of the points". It refers to a specific variety of ventricular tachycardia that exhibits distinct characteristics on the electrocardiogram. The ECG reading in torsades demonstrates a rapid, polymorphic ventricular tachycardia with a characteristic twist of the QRS complex around the isoelectric baseline. P waves are not visible. It is also associated with a fall in arterial blood pressure, which can produce fainting. Although torsade is a rare ventricular arrhythmia, it can degenerate into ventricular fibrillation, which will lead to sudden death in the absence of medical intervention. Torsade de pointes is associated with long QT syndrome, a condition whereby prolonged QT intervals are visible on the ECG. Long QT syndrome [6] can either be inherited as congenital mutations of ion channels carrying the cardiac impulse/action potential or acquired as a result of drugs that block these cardiac ion currents (chapter VI) [11, 12]. Torsades de pointes is associated with bradycardia in the acquired form of long QT syndrome, although it is associated with adrenergic discharge in the congenital form of the long QT syndrome [11] (Fig. **42**).

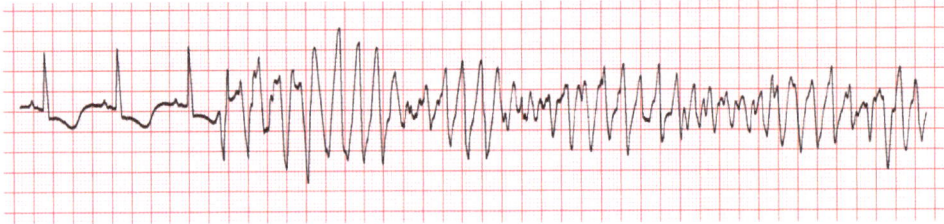

Figure 42: Torsades de pointe caused by acquired long QT syndrome due to antiarrhythmic treatment.

Ventricular Fibrillation

This is a condition in which there is a fast un-coordinated contraction of the cardiac muscle of the ventricles in the heart. It is a chaotic dyssynchronous activity of the heart without identifiable QRS complexes. If the arrhythmia continues for more than a few seconds, blood circulation will cease, and death will occur in a matter of minutes (Fig. **43**).

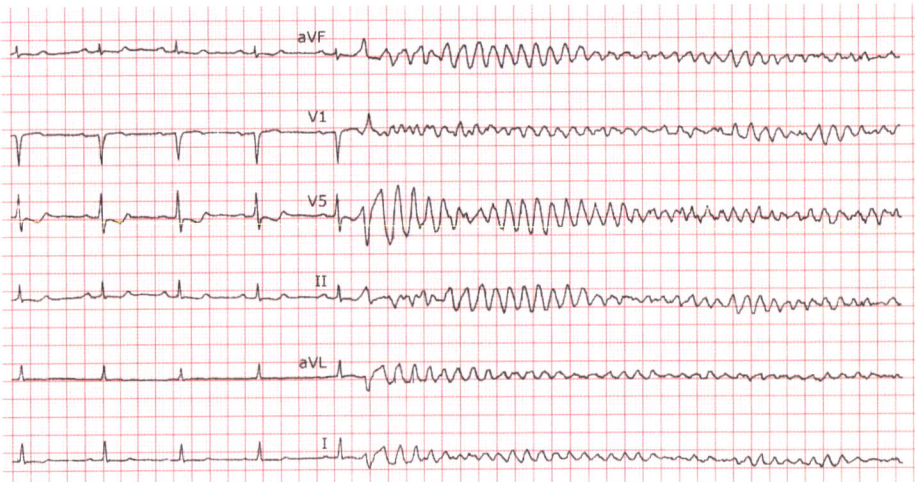

Figure 43: Sinus rhythm on the left portion of the trace. An early ventricular premature contraction (R on T phenomenon) provokes ventricular fibrillation.

ACKNOWLEDGEMENT

Declared none.

CONFLICT OF INTEREST

The author(s) confirm that this chapter content has no conflict of interest.

REFERENCES

[1]   Fisch C: The Electrocardiography of Arrhythmias. Philadelphia, Lea & Febiger, 1990.

[2]   Braunwald's Heart Disease: A Textbook of Cardiovascular Medicine: Elsevier- Saunders, 2011.

[3]   MacFarlane PW, Lawrie TDV (eds): Comprehensive Electrocardiology: Theory and Practice in Health and Disease. Vol 3. New York, Pergamon, 1989.

[4]   Kennedy HL, Goldberger AL, Graboys TB, et al: American College of Cardiology guidelines for training in adult cardiovascular medicine. Task Force 2: Training in electrocardiography, ambulatory electrocardiography, and exercise testing. J Am Coll Cardiol 25:1013, 1995.

[5]   Fisch C, Mandrola JM, Rardon DP: Electrocardiographic manifestations of dual atrioventricular node conduction during sinus rhythm. J Am Coll Cardiol 29:1015-1022, 1997.

[6]   Day CP, McComb JM, Campbell RWF: QT dispersion: An indicator of arrhythmia risk in patients with long QT intervals. Br Heart J 63:342-344, 1990.

[7]   Goldberger AL: Clinical Electrocardiography: A Simplified Approach. 6th ed. St Louis, CV Mosby, 1999.

[8]   Glass L, Mackey MC: From Clocks to Chaos: The Rhythms of Life. Princeton, NJ, Princeton University Press, 1988.

[9]   Chou T-C, Knilans TK: Electrocardiography in Clinical Practice: Adult and Pediatric. 4th ed. Philadelphia, WB Saunders, 1996.

[10]   Schlant RC, Adolph RJ, DiMarco JP, et al: Guidelines for electrocardiography. A report of the American College of Cardiology/American Heart Association Task Force on Assessment of Diagnostic and Therapeutic Cardiovascular Procedures (Committee on Electrocardiography). Circulation 85:1221-1228, 1992.

[11]   Habbab MA, el-Sherif N: TU alternans, long QTU, and torsade de pointes: Clinical and experimental observations. Pacing Clin Electrophysiol 15:916-931, 1992.

[12]   Verrier RL, Nearing BD: Electrophysiologic basis for T wave alternans as an index of vulnerability to ventricular fibrillation. J Cardiovasc Electrophysiol 5:445-461, 1994.

Send Orders of Reprints at reprints@benthamscience.net

CHAPTER 5

Myocardial Ischemia, Myocardial Infarction

Abstract: In this chapter, we address the basic notions of myocardial ischemia and myocardial infarction. Cardiac ischemia changes the electrical activity and the genesis of the action potential and of the resting potential. It can be divided into 3 forms; ischemia, lesion and necrosis. Modification of the QRS complex, the ST segment and T wave is observed. Ischemia is a biochemically reversible anomaly. Moreover, it is mainly ionic, notably potassium disturbances which underlie ST and T wave changes. Lesion is a more severe form of cardiac ischemia but is still reversible, with interstitial oedema and biochemical disturbances. Essentially, it is the ST segment, which is modified, in that it becomes displaced from the isoelectric baseline. The ST segment vector is determined in the same manner as that of the QRS complex: it allows for better localization of the site of the stenosis or obstruction of the culprit artey. The more leads exhibit ST changes, the bigger the territory at risk. A sum total of ST depression or elevation greater than 12 mm in the different leads implies widespread ischemia. The most severe stage of cardiac ischemia is necrosis since there is cellular death with cessation of electrical activity. Neither the action potential nor the resting membrane potential exists anymore and the conduction capability has ceased. The start of depolarisation (QRS) is modified with the apparition of an "electrical hole" (Q waves), which could progress as far as the total disappearance of the positive forces (R waves) and a QS morphology; the necrosis is transmural affecting therefore the full thickness of the myocardium. Acute coronary syndrome includes STEMI and non-STEMI. STEMI (ST Segment Elevation Myocardial Infarction) is the acute coronary syndrome with ST segment elevation and non-STEMI is associated with other ST segment changes (negative T waves or ST segment depression) but not ST segment elevation. Electrocardiographically, the electrical changes recorded in the different territories differ according to the coronary artery involved. There is a good correlation between the ischemic zone and the coronary artery affected. Ischemia is recorded by the electrode "exploring" the territory implicated. Involvement of the right coronary artery gives rise to inferior wall ischemia and this is characterized on the ECG as changes in leads II, III and aVF. Involvement of the left coronary artery gives rise to anterior wall ischemia and this is characterized on the ECG as changes in precordial leads.

Keywords: Myocardial infarction, myocardial ischemia, ST segment Elevation Myocardial Ischemia, non ST segment Elevation Myocardial Ischemia, sub-endocardial myocardial ischemia, sub-epicardial myocardial ischemia, myocardial necrosis, Q wave, ST segment elevation, ST segment depression.

ISCHEMIA

Ischemia is a biochemically reversible anomaly. Moreover, it is mainly ionic, notably potassium disturbances which underlie ST and T wave changes [1,2].

Jean-Jacques Goy, Jean-Christophe Stauffer, Jürg Schlaepfer and Pierre Christeler

Sub-Epicardic Ischemia

Four stages of cardiac repolarisation are observed: 1. The T wave remains positive but begins to appear symmetrical. 2. The T wave is symmetrical with decreased amplitude. 3. The T wave becomes biphasic then negative and asymmetrical. 4. Finally, the T wave is symmetrical and deeply negative.

Sub-Endocardial Ischemia

During an episode of sub-endocardial ischemia, the ischemic zone is within the sub-endocardial layers and repolarisation starts in the superficial layers. Its direction of propagation is not altered, but its depth is reduced. The T wave remains positive but increases in amplitude and symmetry.

In summary: Ischemia is characterized by: 1) A delayed progression of repolarisation (prolonged phase 3). 2) A preserved direction of propagation in sub-endocardial ischemia and 3) A reversed direction of propagation in sub-epicardial ischemia.

LESION

Lesion is a more severe form of cardiac ischemia but is still reversible, with interstitial oedema and biochemical disturbances. Essentially, it is the ST segment, which is modified, in that it becomes displaced from the isoelectric baseline. The ST segment vector is determined in the same manner as that of the QRS complex: it allows for better localization of the site of the stenosis or obstruction of the culprit artey. The more leads exhibit ST changes, the bigger the territory at risk. A sum total of ST depression or elevation greater than 12 mm in the different leads implies widespread ischemia.

Sub-Epicardial Lesion

This affects the superficial layers and is characterized by more marked features on the ECG than with an endocardial lesion. There is ST elevation, which is more prominent if the lesion is transmural. At the outset, the ST elevation starts before the end of the QRS. During the next stage, the ST elevation is more significant and starts in the middle of the QRS. In extreme cases, the QRS acquires the same appearance as the action potential and the ST elevation begins at the peak of the R wave. This appearance is termed Pardee's sign (Fig. **1**).

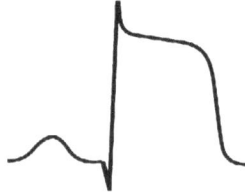

Figure 1: ST elevation during a sub-epicardial lesion, also called Pardee's sign.

Sub-Endocardial Lesion

This involves the deep layers but the electrocardiographic features are often less significant than a sub-epicardial ischemic episode. There is ST depression of > 1 mm, followed by a peaked, symmetrical, positive T wave. This ST depression could be horizontal or downward sloping (Fig. **2**).

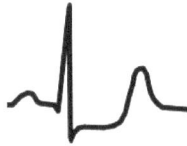

Figure 2: ST depression during a subendocardial lesion.

NECROSIS OR INFARCTION

This is the most severe stage of cardiac ischemia since there is cellular death with cessation of electrical activity. Neither the action potential nor the resting membrane potential exists anymore and the conduction capability has ceased. The start of depolarisation (QRS) is modified with the apparition of an "electrical hole" (Q waves), which could progress as far as the total disappearance of the positive forces (R waves) and a QS morphology; the necrosis is transmural affecting therefore the full thickness of the myocardium. However, the presence of a Q wave does not always signify absence of viable myocardial cells and conversely, the absence of the Q wave does not consistently imply the presence of viable cells.

STEMI AND NON-STEMI

Acute coronary syndrome includes STEMI and non-STEMI. STEMI (ST Segment Elevation Myocardial Infarction) is the acute coronary syndrome with ST segment elevation and non-STEMI is associated with other ST segment changes (negative T waves or ST segment depression) but not ST segment elevation. In both cases, the natural progression could veer towards necrosis or complete resolution of the ischemia without sequelae. It is quite often the case that ischemia, lesion and necrosis are associated and that it is not easy to differentiate between ischemia, ischemia-lesion, *etc.*

In an infarct, there is often a necrosis-lesion-ischemia association. The central necrotic zone is bordered by a lesion zone and surrounded by an ischemic zone. The central zone gives rise to the Q wave, the zone of injury to the ST segment and the ischemic zone to the T wave changes. There is not always a good correlation between electrical activity and myocardial function. It is possible to have good left ventricular function after an infarct even though the electrical activity suggests widespread necrosis. The reverse is also true [3].

Consequences

1. The Q wave is a sign of necrosis (8). A significant Q wave lasts > 40 ms with an amplitude of > 25 % of the R wave.

2. The depth of the Q wave correlates with the thickness of the necrosis.

3. The residual R wave amplitude corresponds to the remaining healthy myocardium.

ISCHEMIA LOCALIZATION

Electrocardiographically, the electrical changes recorded in the different territories differ according to the coronary artery involved. There is a good correlation between the ischemic zone and the coronary artery affected. Ischemia is recorded by the electrode "exploring" the territory implicated. Involvement of the right coronary artery gives rise to inferior wall ischemia and this is characterized on the ECG as changes in leads II, III and aVF [4-7].

Inferior Ischemia (Fig. 3)

> - Sub-epicardial: negative T waves in II, III and aVF.
>
> - Sub-endocardial: positive and large T waves in II, III and aVF.

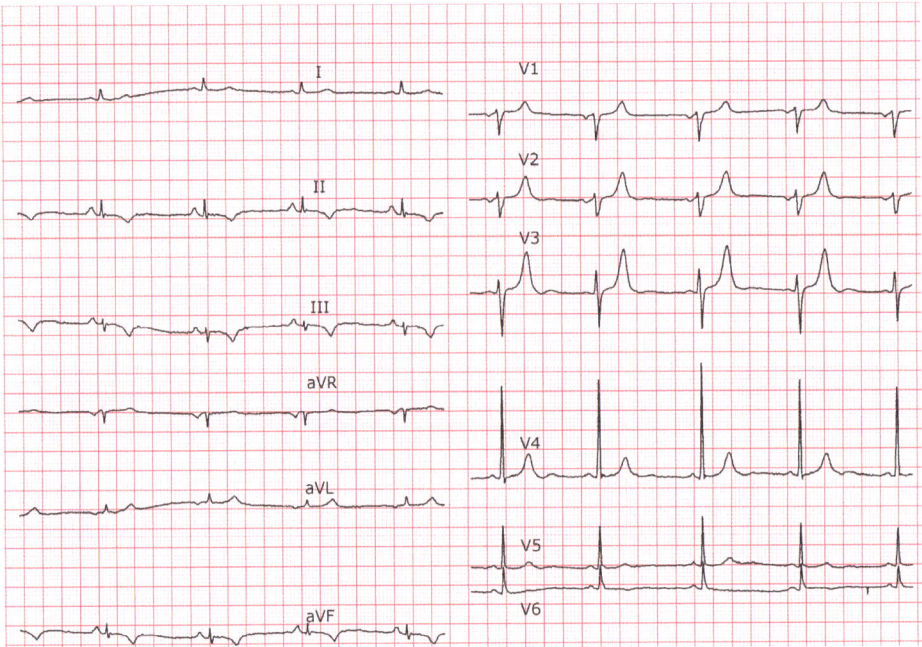

Figure 3: Inferior sub-endocardial ischemia. The very peaked T waves in V2 and V3 are a mirror image of this ischemia.

Antero-Septal Ischemia (Figs. 4 and 5)

> - Sub-epicardial: flat T waves, biphasic or negative in V1, V2, V3 and sometimes V4.
>
> - Sub-endocardial: positive peaked T waves, with increased amplitude and in V1, V2, V3 and sometimes V4.

Anterior Ischemia (Fig. 6)

> - Sub-epicardial: negative T waves from V1 to V5 or V6.
>
> - Sub-endocardial: very positive and peaked T waves from V1 to V5 or even V6.

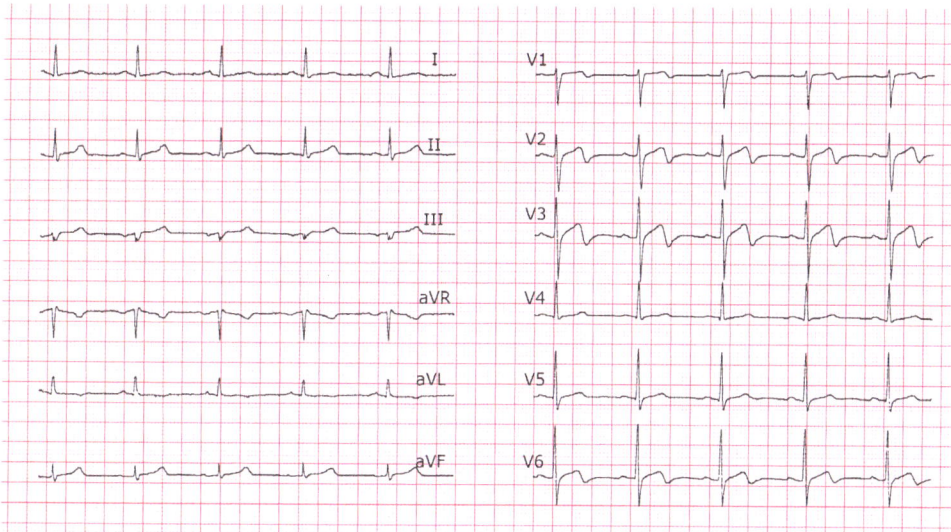

Figure 4: Antero-septal sub-epicardial ischemia is characterized by biphasic T waves from V1 to V3.

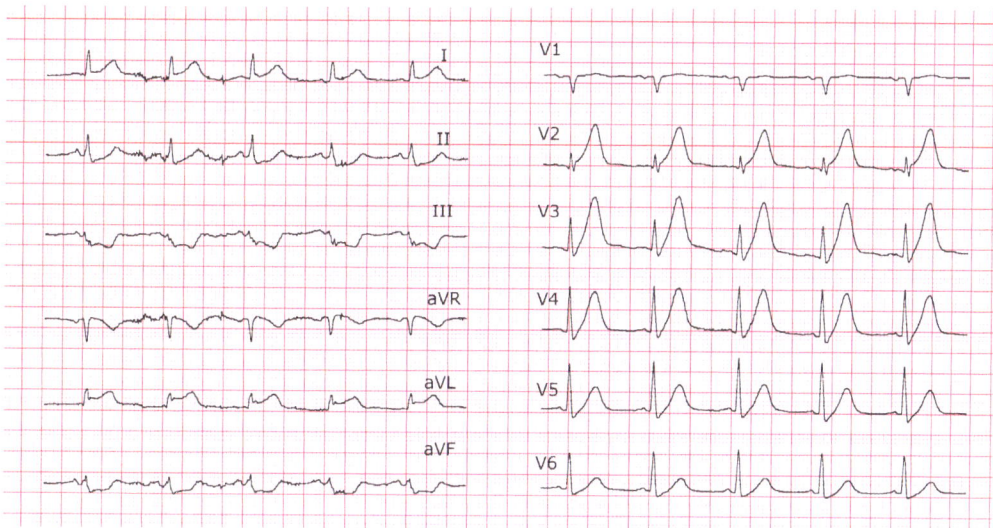

Figure 5: Anterior sub-endocardial ischemia-lesion extending from V2 to V5. The ST segment elevation in I and aVL is due to a lateral lesion picture.

Lateral Ischemia (Fig. 7)

- Sub-epicardial: Biphasic flat or inverted T wave in I, aVL, V5, V6.

- Sub-endocardial: Tall peaked symmetrical T wave, positive in I, aVL, V5 and V6.

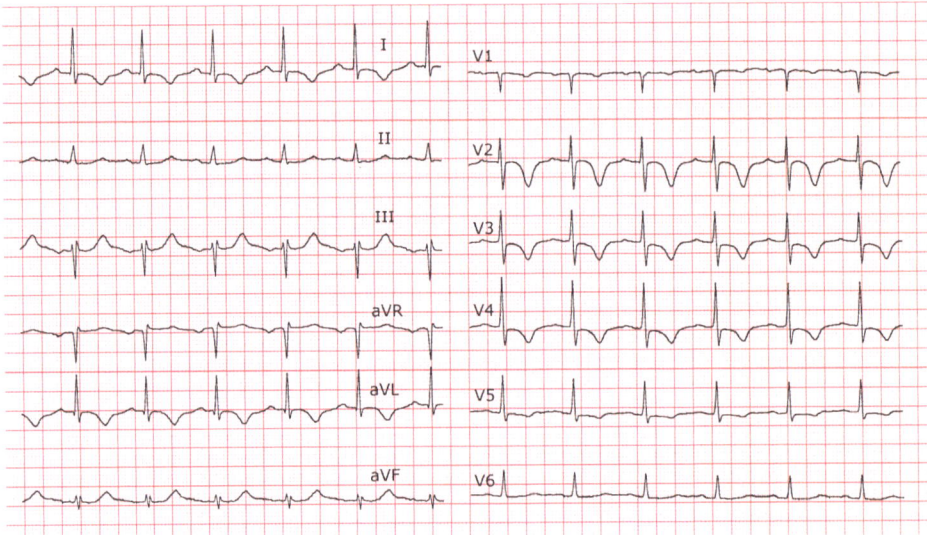

Figure 6: Sub-epicardial antero-septal and lateral ischemia or lesion with abnormal ST segment from V2 to V5 and in I and aVL.

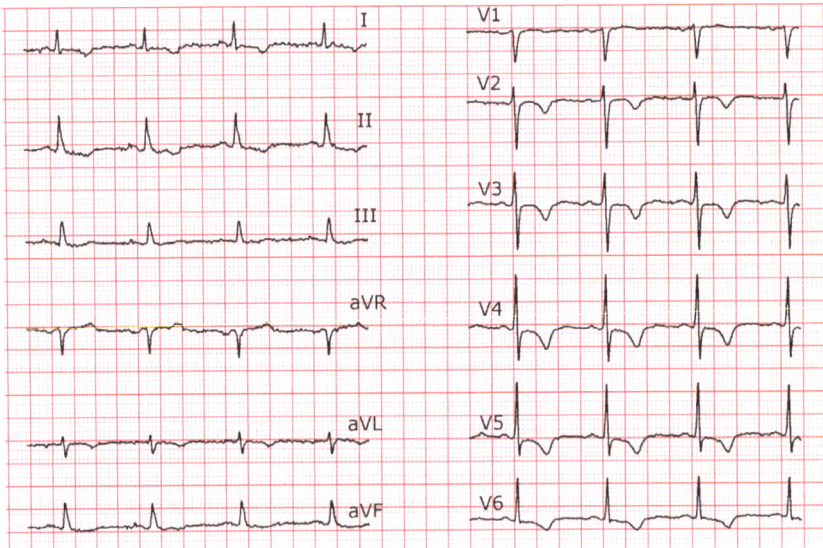

Figure 7: Widespread anterior sub-epicardial ischemia with lateral extension (T waves negative from V2 to V6 and in I and aVL).

Inferior Lesion (Fig. 8)

- Sub-epicardial: ST segment elevation in II, III and aVF.

- Sub-endocardial: ST depression in II, III and aVF.

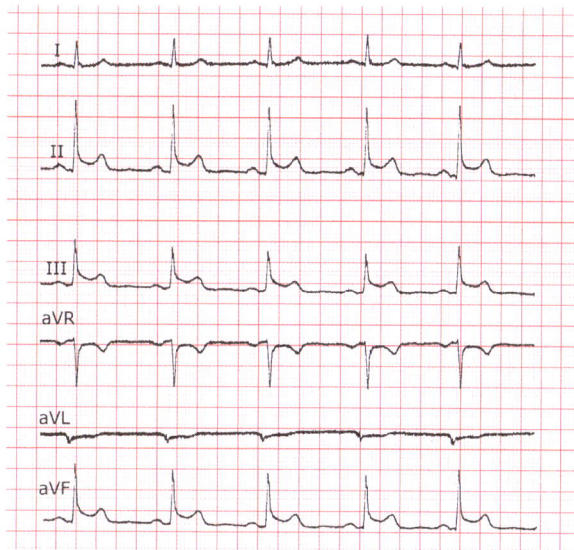

Figure 8: Inferior lesion characterized by ST segment elevation in leads II, III and aVF.

Antero-Septal Lesion (Fig. 9)

- Sub-epicardial: ST segment elevation in V1, V2, V3, sometimes V4.

- Sub-endocardial: ST segment depression in V1, V2, V3, sometimes V4.

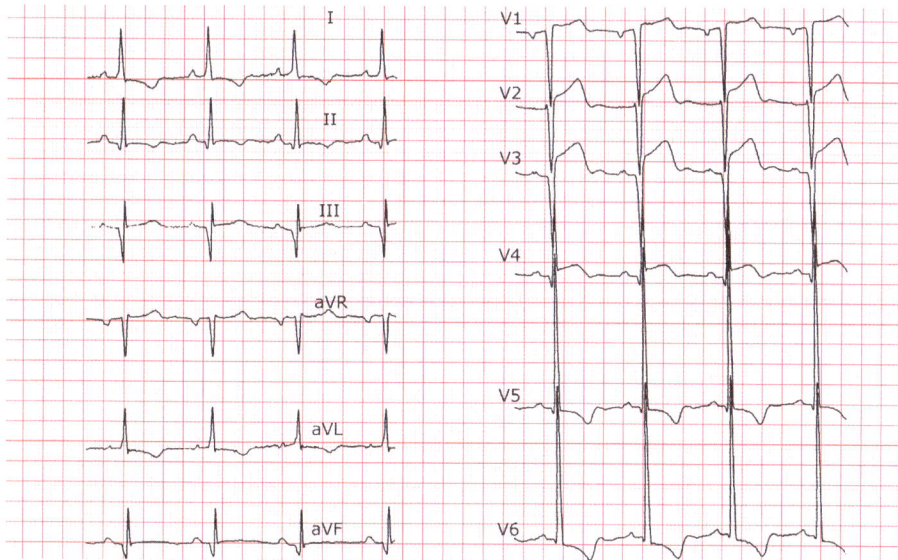

Figure 9: Antero-septal lesion picture with an old inferior infarct (Q wave in III and aVF). The Q wave in V3 is a sign of an anterior infarct as well as a lesion picture.

Anterior Lesion (Fig. 10)

- Sub-epicardial: ST elevation from V1 to V6.

- Sub-endocardial: ST depression from V1 to V6.

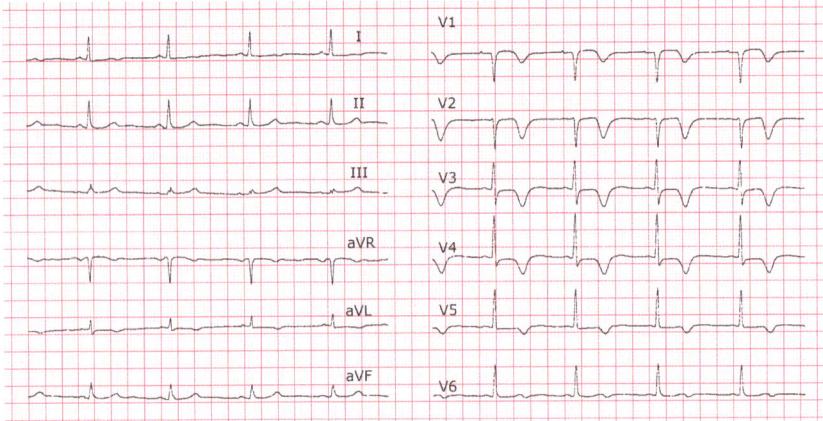

Figure 10: Deep negative T waves from V1 to V5 corresponding to a widespread anterior sub-epicardial ischemia.

Lateral Lesion (Fig. 11)

- Sub-epicardial: ST elevation in I, aVL, V5, V6.

- Sub-endocardial: ST depression in I, aVL, V5, V6.

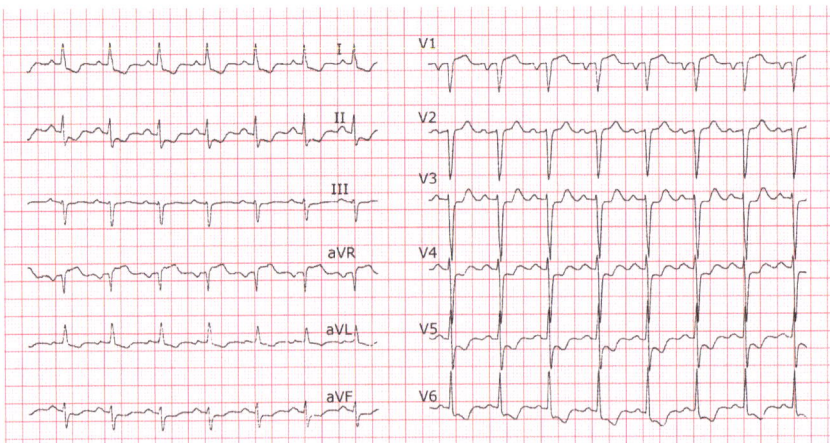

Figure 11: Picture of widespread anterior and lateral sub-epicardial lesion due to a very proximal coronary lesion characterized by ST depression from V3 to V6, in I, II, III, aVF and aVL. The ST elevation in V1 and aVR is suspicious of a left main stem lesion or the equivalent of a left main stem.

The significance of the sum of the recorded ST depression in the different leads has a prognostic value. There is a correlation between the number of leads with ST depression and the extent and severity of the coronary disease. ST depression in at least 8 leads associated with ST elevation in V1 and aVR is suggestive of severe 3 vessel disease or a stenosis of the left main stem.

ST Segment Depression in the Precordial Leads

As with the QRS complex, ST elevation can be represented by a vector. The direction of this vector can be used to precisely localize the site of occlusion of the left anterior descending (LAD) artery, responsible for anterior infarcts. It is important to bear in mind that the distribution of the branches of the LAD is variable, which explains the great diversity of ECGs of anterior infarction [4-6].

1. If the occlusion is very proximal: there is ST segment elevation from V1 to V4, in aVR and aVL, ST depression in II, III, aVF, isoelectric ST segment or depression in V5-V6.

2. If the occlusion is located after the first septal but before the first diagonal branch: there is ST elevation from V2 to V5, in I and aVL, ST depression in III (Fig. **12**).

3. If the occlusion is distal to the first diagonal but proximal to the first septal branch: there is ST elevation from V1 to V5, in III, aVR, ST depression in I and aVL.

4. If the occlusion is distal to the first septal and the first diagonal: there is ST elevation from V2 to V6, in II, III, aVF (II > III), ST depression in aVR.

ST Depression in the Inferior Leads

ST depression in the inferior leads could be secondary to disease in the right coronary artery or the circumflex artery [7-9].

With right coronary disease, the ST depression in lead III is more marked than in lead II; it is often accompanied by ST depression in lead I. If the occlusion is proximal (proximal to the right marginal branches) there is ST elevation (> 1mm) in V4R with a positive T wave [10]. This reflects involvement of the right ventricle; if the lesion is distal, the ST segment is isoelectric and the T wave is positive in V4R [11].

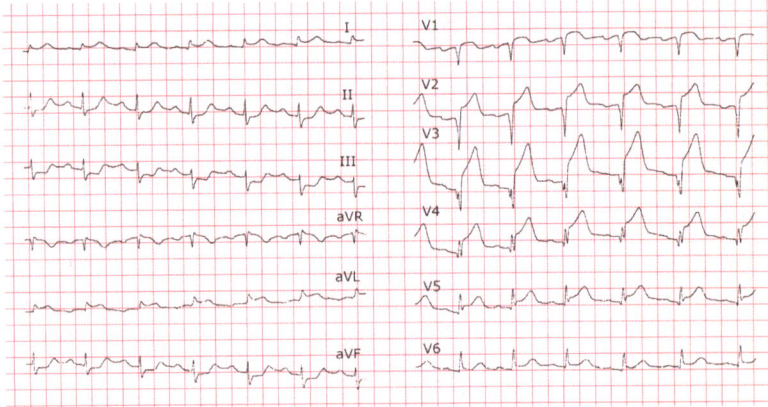

Figure 12: Anterior lesion picture. The occlusion is probably located after the first septal but before the first diagonal.

In the case of circumflex artery occlusions, ST elevation in II is more marked than in III; the ST segment is isoelectric or elevated in I, isoelectric or negative with negative T wave in V4R (Fig. **13**).

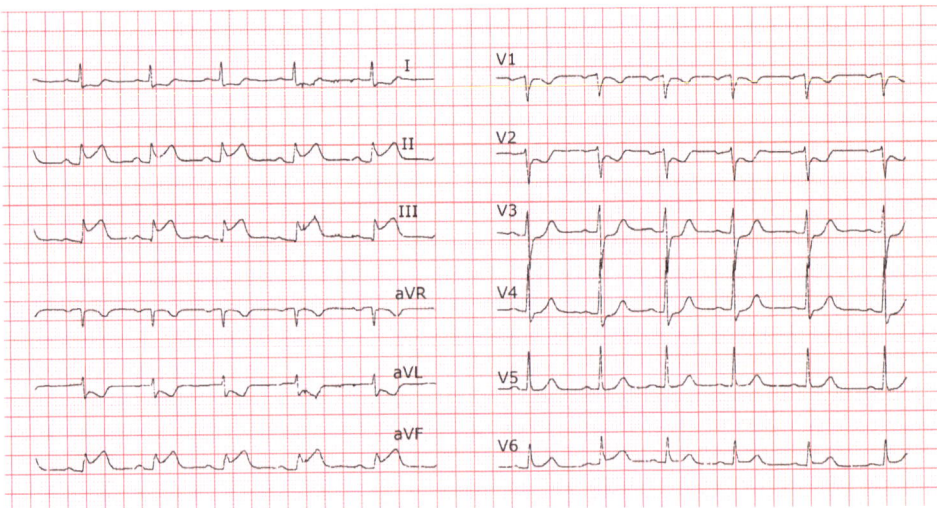

Figure 13: Sinus rhythm with ST elevation in II, III and aVF. This ST elevation is more marked in III and corresponds to inferior ischemia due to right coronary occlusion.

If there is a "posterior" extension, there will be ST depression in the chest leads; if the extension is lateral, there will be ST elevation in I, aVL, V5, V6.

NECROSIS

The electrocardiographic picture depends on the territory affected and Q waves as previously mentioned, are seen in these territories [12-14]:

1. Widespread anterior necrosis: presence of necrosis waves (QS or QR) in all the precordial leads from V1 to V6, in I and aVL (4) (Fig. **14**).

2. Antero-septal necrosis: QS from V1 to V3 sometimes in V4. The Q wave is explained by the disappearance of the r wave, which represents initial septal activation.

3. Apical necrosis: Q waves appear in V3, V4.

4. Lateral necrosis: QS or QR in V5, V6, I and aVL is observed. The usual morphology is of the type QR or qR due to the fact that there is generally some healthy myocardial tissue adjacent to the zone of necrosis. In some cases, the q wave is small and it is therefore not easy to categorically assure oneself of the existence of the infarct.

5. Inferior necrosis: QS or qR in II, III and aVF (Figs. **15** and **16**). If a Q wave is present in only one of these leads, the ECG should be repeated in maximal inspiration because some q waves (especially in lead III) could be "positional". This is due to changes in the position of the heart within the chest cavity, linked to the respiratory cycle.

Widespread anterior necrosis: presence of necosis waves (QS or QR) in all the precordial leads from V1 to V6 and in I and aVL (Fig. **14**).

"Posterior" necrosis: these necrosis are often associated with inferior necrosis. In cases where they are isolated, there is a tall R wave in V1. During an inferior necrosis, in addition to a standard ECG, a recording of right precordial leads should also be performed. This could show ST changes (during the first 12 hours of an infarct) at the time of right ventricular ischemia (V4 R) (Fig. **17**).

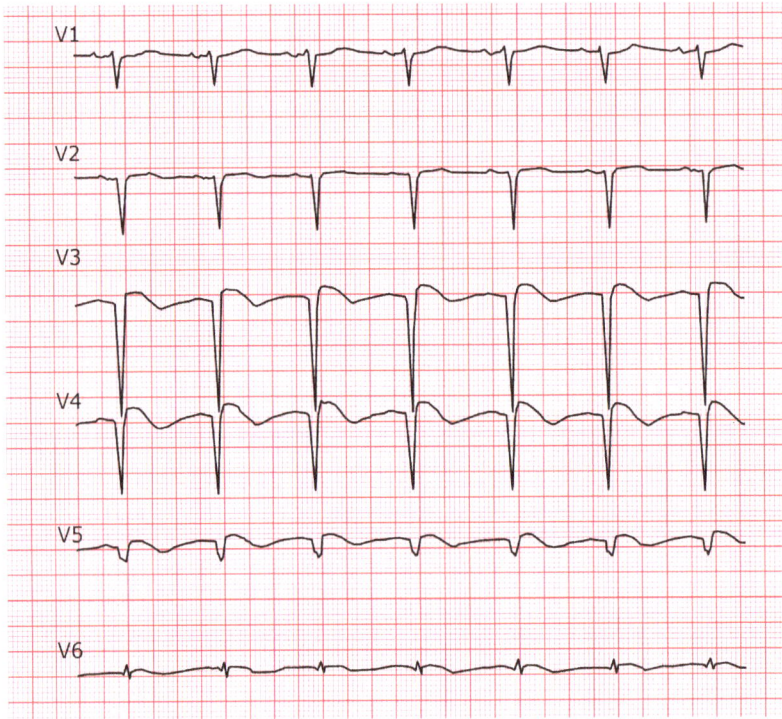

Figure 14: Partial recording of the precordial leads demonstrating an anterior necrosis picture Q waves from V2 to V5. Persistent ST elevation is compatible with an aneurysm or dyskinesia of the anterior wall.

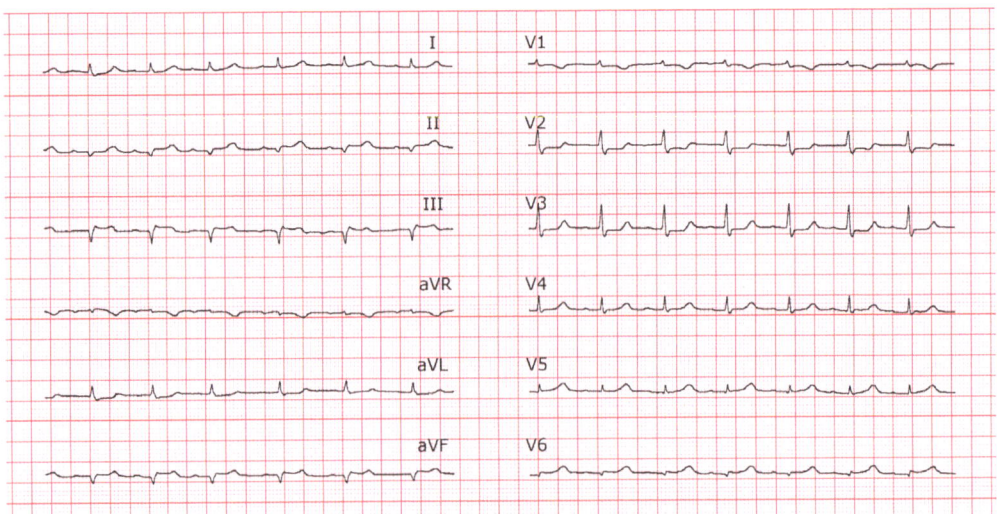

Figure 15: Q waves in II, III and aVF associated with ST elevation in the same leads corresponding to an inferior necrosis. The R wave in V1 is due to a posterior extension of the necrosis.

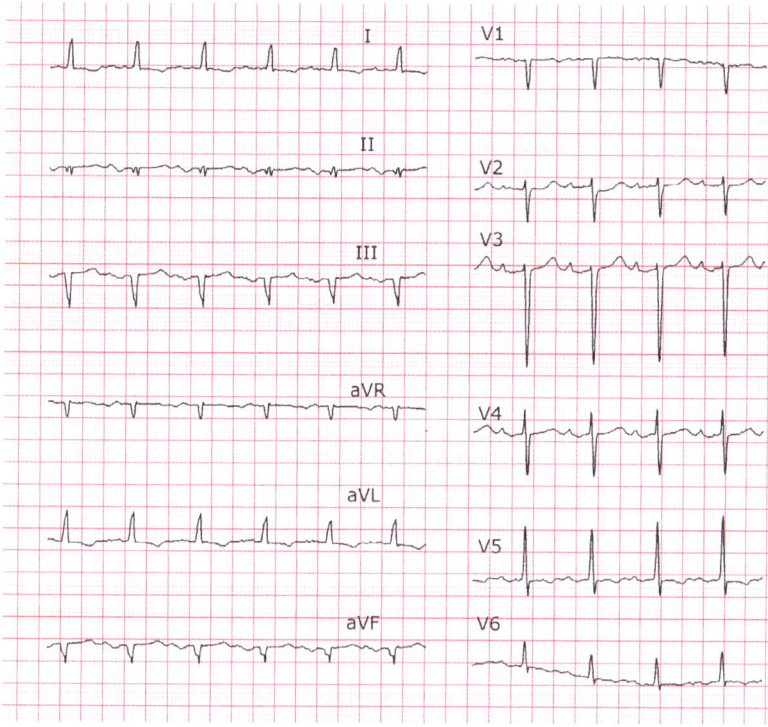

Figure 16: Inferior necrosis with Q waves in II, III and aVF. The negative T waves in I, aVL and V6 are as a result of a lateral sub-epicardial ischemia.

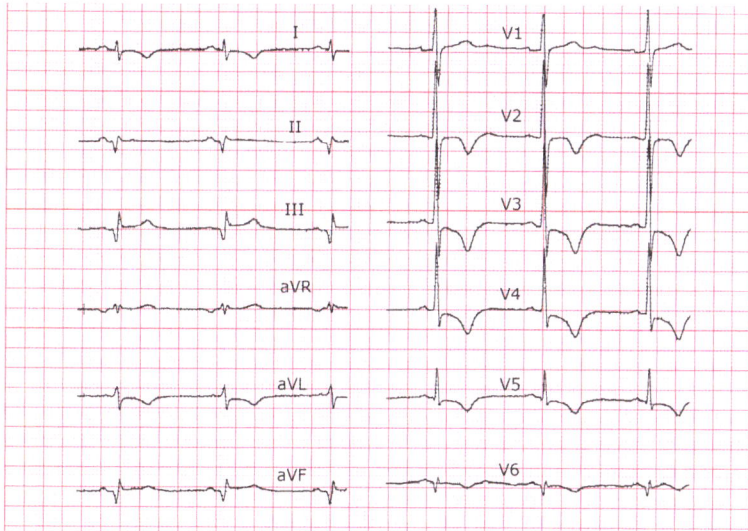

Figure 17: Inferior necrosis with Q waves in II, III and aVF. The Q wave in V6 is due to a lateral extension of the necrosis and the tall R wave in V1 to a posterior extension. The negative T waves from V2 to V5 are due to an anterior sub-epicardial ischemia.

TAKO-TSUBO SYNDROME

This is quite a rare syndrome which is seen more frequently in middle age women (after the menopause). It is characterized by acute coronary syndrome picture with ischemic ST changes, even including ST elevation in the precordial leads. The symptoms, which are basically typical anginal pain, are generally induced by extreme stress. The coronary vessels are normal but at left ventriculogram, there is an apico-anterior akinesia, which regresses within 2-3 months (Fig. **18**).

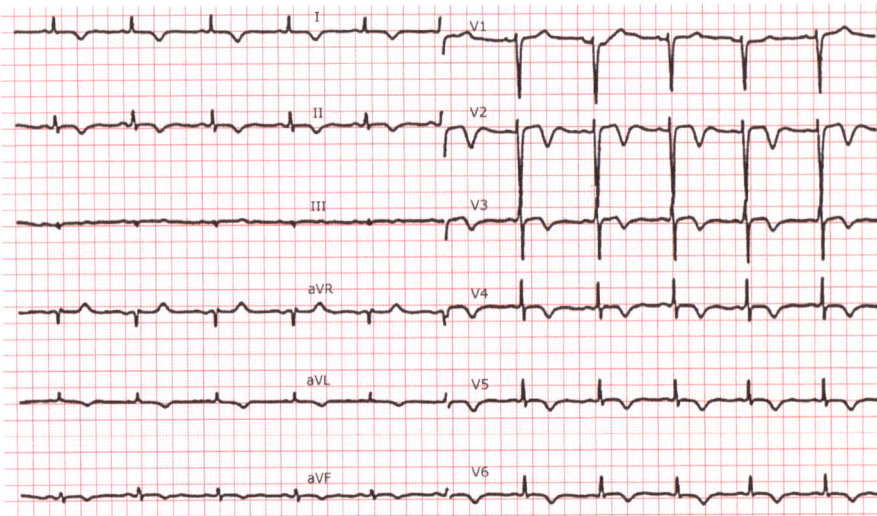

Figure 18: Anterior ischemic picture as would be seen in a case of Tako-Tsubo syndrome.

ACKNOWLEDGEMENT

Declared none.

CONFLICT OF INTEREST

The author(s) confirm that this chapter content has no conflict of interest.

REFERENCES

[1]   Goldberger AL: Myocardial Infarction: Electrocardiographic Differential Diagnosis. 4th ed. St Louis, Mosby-Year Book, 1991.
[2]   Mirvis DM: Electrocardiography: A Physiologic Approach. St Louis, Mosby-Year Book, 1993.

[3]   Clements IP (ed): The Electrocardiogram in Acute Myocardial Infarction. Armonk, NY, Futura, 1998.

[4]   Engelen DJ, Gorgels AP, Cheriex EC, et al: Value of the electrocardiogram in localizing the occlusion site in the left anterior descending coronary artery in acute anterior myocardial infarction. J Am Coll Cardiol 34:389-395, 1999.

[5]   Kontos MC, Desai PV, Jesse RL, et al: Usefulness of the admission electrocardiogram for identifying the infarct-related artery in inferior wall acute myocardial infarction. Am J Cardiol 79:182-184, 1997.

[6]   Mirvis DM, Ingram LA, Ramanathan KB, et al: R and S wave changes produced by experimental nontransmural and transmural myocardial infarction. J Am Coll Cardiol 8:675-681, 1986.

[7]   Arbane M, Goy JJ: Prediction of the site of total occlusion in the left anterior descending coronary artery using admission electrocardiogram in anterior wall acute myocardial infarction. Am J Cardiol 85:487-491, 2000.

[8]   Kosuge M, Kimura K, Ishikawa T, et al: New electrocardiographic criteria for predicting the site of coronary artery occlusion in inferior wall acute myocardial infarction. Am J Cardiol 82:1318-1322, 1998.

[9]   Herz I, Assali AR, Adler Y, et al: New electrocardiographic criteria for predicting either the right or left circumflex artery as the culprit coronary artery in inferior wall acute myocardial infarction. Am J Cardiol 80:1343-1345, 1997.

[10]   Assali AR, Sclarovsky S, Herz I, et al: Comparison of patients with inferior wall acute myocardial infarction with versus without ST-segment elevation in leads V5 and V6 . Am J Cardiol 81:81-83, 1998.

[11]   Kinch JW, Ryan TJ: Right ventricular infarction. N Engl J Med 330:1211, 1994.

[12]   Macfarlane PW, Lawrie TDV: Comprehensive Electrocardiography. New York, Pergamon, 1989.

[13]   Braunwald's Heart Disease : A Textbook of Cardiovascular Medicine: Elsevier- Saunders, 2011.

[14]   Wong ND, Levy D, Kannel WB: Prognostic significance of the electrocardiogram after Q wave myocardial infarction. The Framingham Study. Circulation 81:780-789, 1990.

Send Orders of Reprints at reprints@benthamscience.net

CHAPTER 6

Differential Diagnosis of Cardiac Ischemia

Abstract: In this chapter, we address the basic notions of the differential diagnosis of cardiac ischemia. Hypertrophic obstructive cardiomyopathy or HOCM is characterized on the electrocardiogram by Q waves in the inferior leads and negative T waves from V2 to V5 which is difficult to distinguish from classical ischemia due to coronary pathology.The electrocardiographic abnormalities of pericarditis are non specific and sometimes difficult to distinguish from ischemia. They are typically recognized by PR segment depression, present in the majority of the leads. The repolarisation abnormalities it causes are very similar to those of ischemia-lesion; primarily, the ST segment is elevated, with an inferior convexity, the so-called "camel hump" appearance. This segment progressively returns to the isoelectric line in the same time it takes for the amplitude of the T wave to fall, and in the end becomes negative. In V5, the amplitude of the ST elevation, compared to the amplitude of the T wave is > 0.25: a ratio < 0.25 favours early repolarisation. The electrical features of pericarditis are reputed to be diffuse, but in reality are not always so. Occasionally, acute pericarditis is the cause of an arrhythmia, almost always supraventricular (atrial fibrillation). However, there is never a pathological Q wave of necrosis. Moreover, the changes are generally diffuse and widespread without systemization of coronary abnormalities. The electrocardiographic features of pulmonary embolism are not specific: on the background of preexisting right bundle branch block, the Q waves in III and QS in V1 could be due to an inferior or an antero-septal infarct respectively. In the same vein, the raised ST segment in V1 could also be an antero-septal ischemia-lesion picture. Chatterjee phenomenon is a T wave inversion, often deep, which occurs after a period of abnormal ventricular activation (broad QRS), notably ventricular tachycardia, intermittent left bundle branch block or preexcitation, or even intermittent ventricular pacing. Early repolarisation causes in leads V2 to V5, a raised J-point and ST segment, as well as an increase in the amplitude of a symmetrical T wave, as would be expected for an ischemia-lesion but the J-point remains prominent and the convexity of the ST is inferior and not superior. Brugada syndrome is not a conduction abnormality but deserves a mention under the heading of right bundle branch block as it can mimic some aspects, notably changes in the terminal phase. There are 3 types of changes in V1 and V2 and rarely in V3. In all 3 types the J-point is raised at least 2 mm.

Keywords: Pericarditis, hypertrophic cardiomyopathy, Chatterjee phenomenon, early repolarization, Brugada syndrome, PR segment depression, ST segment elevation, pulmonary embolism, rigth ventricular dilatation.

HYPERTROPHIC OBSTRUCTIVE CARDIOMYOPATHY

Classically, hypertrophic obstructive cardiomyopathy or HOCM is characterized on the electrocardiogram by Q waves in the inferior leads and negative T waves

Jean-Jacques Goy, Jean-Christophe Stauffer, Jürg Schlaepfer and Pierre Christeler

from V2 to V5 which is difficult to distinguish from classical ischemia due to coronary pathology [1, 2] (Fig. **1**).

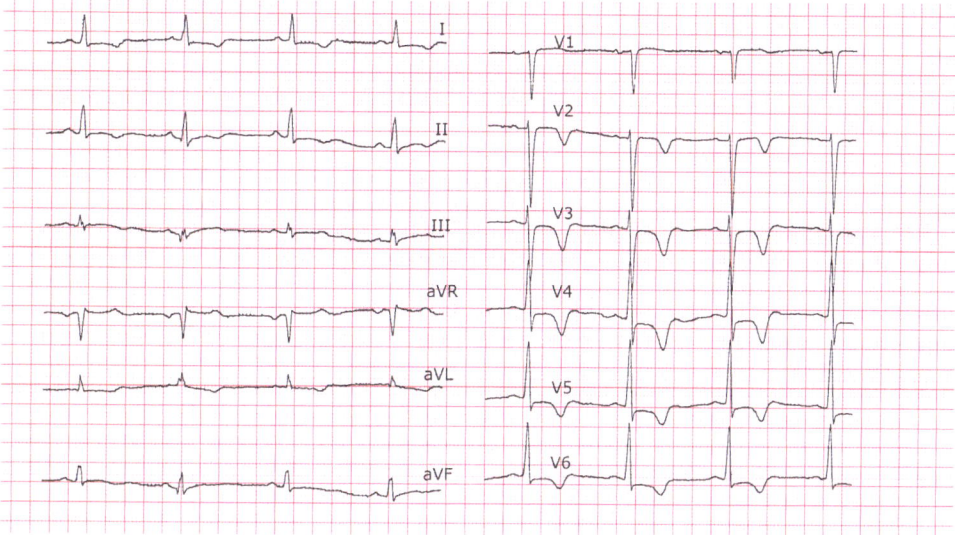

Figure 1: Sinus rhythm with negative T waves from V2 to V6, in lead I and aVL, in a patient with HOCM but no coronary disease.

ACUTE PERICARDITIS

The electrocardiographic abnormalities of pericarditis are non specific and sometimes difficult to distinguish from ischemia. They are typically recognized by PR segment depression, present in the majority of the leads. The repolarisation abnormalities it causes are very similar to those of ischemia-lesion; primarily, the ST segment is elevated, with an inferior convexity, the so-called "camel hump" appearance. This segment progressively returns to the isoelectric line in the same time it takes for the amplitude of the T wave to fall, and in the end becomes negative. In V5, the amplitude of the ST elevation, compared to the amplitude of the T wave is > 0.25: a ratio < 0.25 favours early repolarisation. The electrical features of pericarditis are reputed to be diffused, but in reality are not always so. Occasionally, acute pericarditis is the cause of an arrhythmia, almost always supraventricular (atrial fibrillation). However, there is never a pathological Q wave of necrosis. Moreover, the changes are generally diffused and widespread without systemization of coronary abnormalities. There are generally 4 phases during the natural progression of pericarditis [3, 4]:

1. Diffuse concave ST elevation different from that of myocardial infarction, the so-called "saddleback" appearance.

2. The ST elevation reduces with a return to the isoelectric line and a biphasic or flattened morphology.

3. T wave inversion the depth of which is not very significant, negative and symmetrical appearance, quite similar to T wave inversion of ischemic origin.

4. A chronic phase with progressive normalization of the T wave which become less negative and reassumes its normal positive shape.

In addition, there is PR segment depression in the majority of leads except in aVR and V1 where the PR is elevated. The trace below (Fig. **2**) is one such example where all the abnormalities cited above are shown.

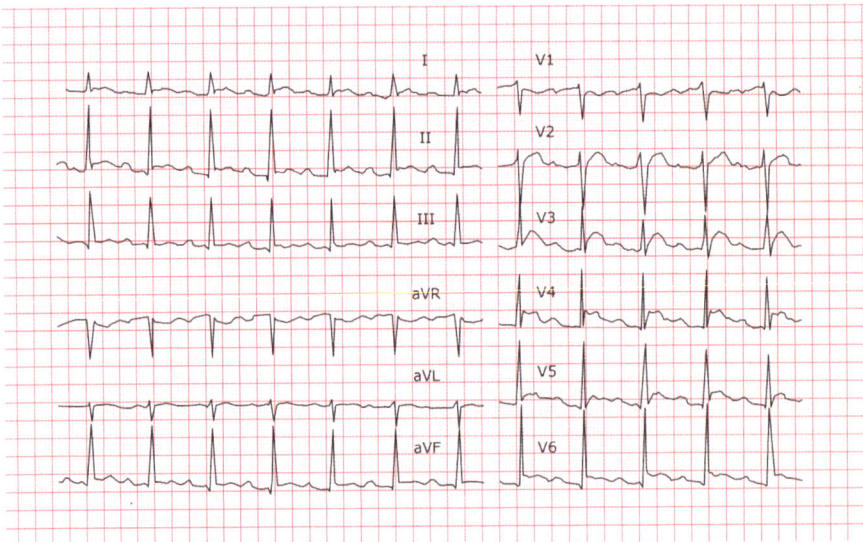

Figure 2: Diffused ST elevation, with depression of the PR segment in II and elevation in aVR and V1 in the context of acute pericarditis.

A pericardial effusion, if it is large, reduces that amplitude of all the QRS complexes. There is sometimes alternans of the QRS complexes (alternating amplitude from one complex to the next).

It is common to find it difficult to choose between an infarct and pericarditis especially at the beginning of disease evolution, when the Q wave is not yet apparent in the case of infarct.

PULMONARY EMBOLISM

Right ventricular dilatation causes stretching of the right branch of the His bundle, which results in a sudden incomplete right bundle branch block, indeed complete block if the embolus cuts off more than 50% of the pulmonary circulation. An embolus is suspected if in V1, the terminal phase takes on an atypical appearance of ST elevation followed by a symmetrical and negative T wave. This phenomenon becomes more marked when the QRS, principally triphasique with an R', acquires a qR appearance, indeed QS. The electrical axis of the heart is displaced towards the right without necessarily exceeding + 90°. Ventricular dilatation also leads to a clockwise rotation of the heart around its cranio-caudal axis as attested by an S1q3T3 appearance (T wave - in III) and in the precordial leads by a displacement of the zone of transition. The zone of transition corresponds to a precordial lead (normally V3) where the amplitude of the R wave is closest to that of the S wave, towards the left (Fig. **3**).

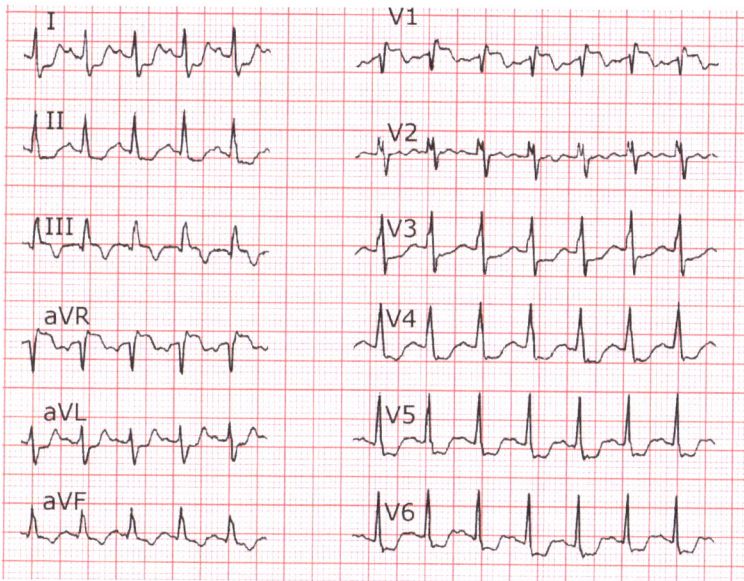

Figure 3: ECG recorded during the course of a pulmonary embolus with the classic signs, namely: S1 et q3 waves with negative T waves in III and ST elevation in V1.

The electrocardiographic features of pulmonary embolism are not specific: on the background of preexisting right bundle branch block, the Q waves in III and QS in V1 could be due to an inferior or an antero-septal infarct, respectively. In the same vein, the raised ST segment in V1 could also be an antero-septal ischemia-lesion picture [5,6].

CHATTERJEE PHENOMENON

Chatterjee phenomenon is a T wave inversion, often deep, which occurs after a period of abnormal ventricular activation (broad QRS), notably ventricular tachycardia, intermittent left bundle branch block or preexcitation, or even intermittent ventricular pacing. The phenomenon can last several days (Fig. **4**) [7].

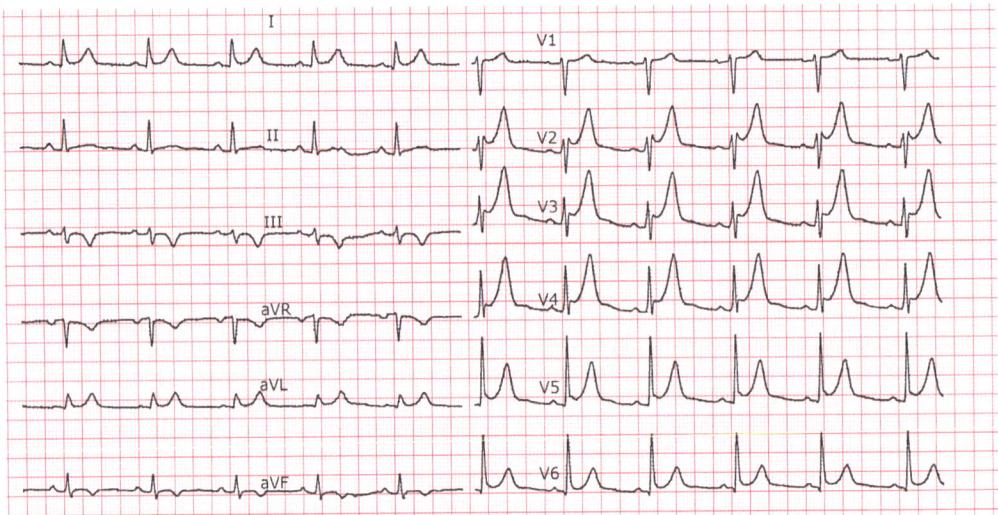

Figure 4: Sinus rhythm recorded hours after ablation of an accessory pathway. The T waves, in III and aVF, correspond to Chatterjee phenomenon, which is due to a memory effect of the preexcitation. It is caused by the change in depolarisation and hence the repolarisation.

EARLY REPOLARISATION

Early repolarisation causes in leads V2 to V5, a raised J-point and ST segment, as well as an increase in the amplitude of a symmetrical T wave, as would be expected for an ischemia-lesion but the J-point remains prominent and the convexity of the ST is inferior and not superior. The descending phase of the R wave is slowed immediately prior to the J point, a small irregularity. In V5, the ratio of ST elevation (in mm) to that of the T wave (in mm) is less than 0.25, whilst for pericarditis it is greater than 0.25. This anomaly is frequently observed in young black people. The 4 characteristics of early repolarisation are [8, 9] (Fig. **5**):

1. ST elevation starting at the J-point, of up to 1 to 4 mm

2. Upward ST segment concavity ("saddleback" appearance)

3. Little notch or slowing of the descending slope of the R wave;

4. Tall symmetrical T wave.

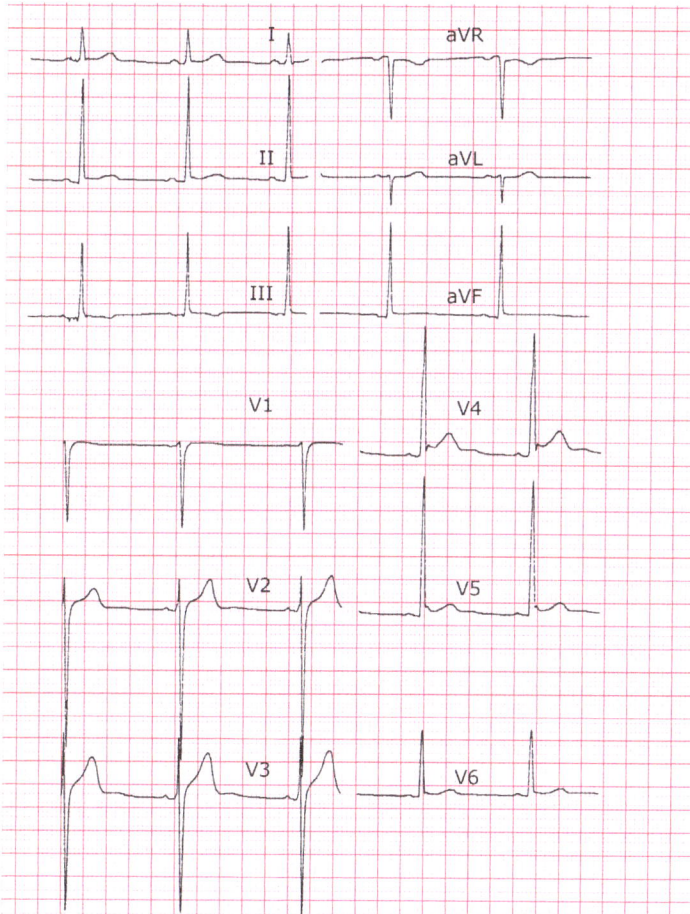

Figure 5: ECG of a young patient of 19 years with typical changes of early repolarisation.

BRUGADA SYNDROME

Brugada syndrome is not a conduction abnormality but deserves a mention under the heading of right bundle branch block as it can mimic some aspects, notably changes in the terminal phase. There are 3 types of changes in V1 and V2 and rarely in V3. In all 3 types the J-point is raised at least 2 mm [10, 11].

1. The descending part of the ST segment is oblique with a negative T wave. This repolarisation abnormality is not always evident (Fig. **6**).

2. The ST segment takes on a "saddleback" appearance, with an elevation of ≤ 1 mm, followed by a positive or biphasic T wave.

3. The ST segment has a saddleback appearance. It is raised by < 1 mm with a positive T wave.

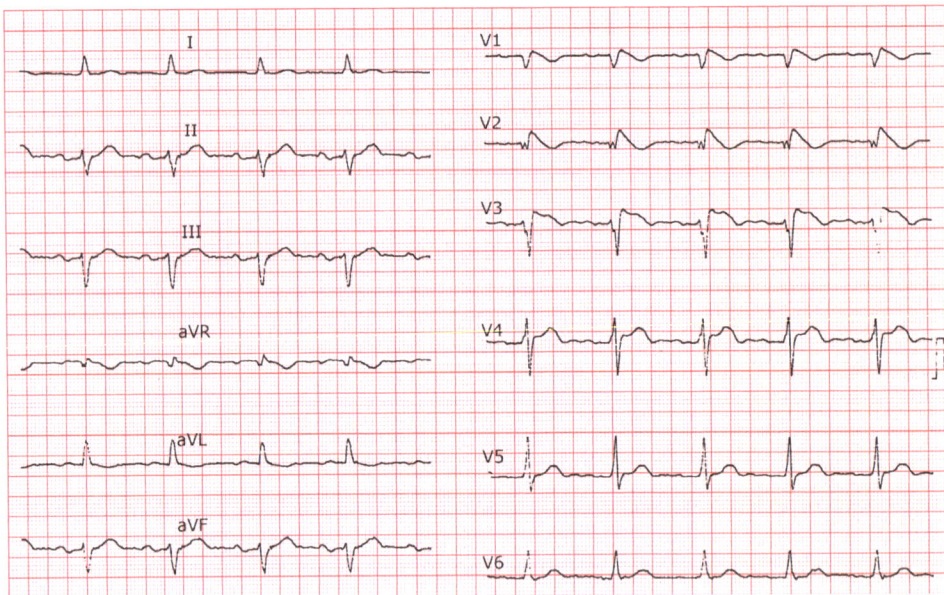

Figure 6: Abnormalities of the QRS in V1, V2, V3 with ST segment elevation and oblique descent typical of Brugada syndrome type 1.

ACKNOWLEDGEMENT

Declared none.

CONFLICT OF INTEREST

The author(s) confirm that this chapter content has no conflict of interest.

REFERENCES

[1]   Maron BJ. Q waves in hypertrophic cardiomyopathy: A reassessment. J Am Coll Cardiol 16:375-376, 1990.

[2]   Usui M, Inoue H, Suzuki J, *et al.* Relationship between distribution of hypertrophic and electrocardiographic changes in hypertrophic cardiomyopathy. Am Heart J 126:177-183, 1993.

[3]   Bonnefoy E, Godon P, Kirkorian G, *et al.* Serum cardiac troponin I and ST-segment elevation in patients with acute pericarditis [Comment] Eur Heart J 21:832-836, 2000.

[4]   Baljepally R, Spodick DH: PR-segment deviation as the initial electrocardiographic response in acute pericarditis. Am J Cardiol 81:1505-1506, 1998.

[5]   Tighe DA, Chung EK, Park CH: Electric alternans associated with acute pulmonary embolism. Am Heart J 128:188-190, 1994.

[6]   Sreeram N, Cheriex EC, Smeets JL, *et al.* Value of the 12-lead electrocardiogram at hospital admission in the diagnosis of pulmonary embolism. Am J Cardiol 73:298-303, 1994.

[7]   Geller JC, Rosen MR: Persistent T-wave changes after alteration of the ventricular activation sequence: New insights into cellular mechanisms of 'cardiac memory.' Circulation 88:1811-1819, 1993.

[8]   Haydar ZR, Brantley DA, Gittings NS, *et al.* Early repolarization: An electrocardiographic predictor of enhanced aerobic fitness. Am J Cardiol 85:264-266, 2000.

[9]   Mehta M, Jain AC, Mehta A: Early repolarization. Clin Cardiol 27:59-65, 1999

[10]   Brugada P, Brugada J: Right bundle branch block, persistent ST segment elevation and sudden cardiac death: A distinct clinical and electrocardiographic syndrome. A multicenter report. J Am Coll Cardiol 20:1391-1396, 1992.

[11]   Tada H, Nogami A, Shimizu W, *et al.* ST segment and T wave alternans in a patient with Brugada syndrome. Pacing Clin Electrophysiol 23:413-415, 2000.

Send Orders of Reprints at reprints@benthamscience.net

Electrocardiography (ECG), 2013, 124-132

CHAPTER 7

Hypertrophy

Abstract: In this chapter, we address the basic notions of cardiac chambers hypertrophy. Hypertrophy of the left ventricle causes a significant increase in the height and depth of the QRS complex. The thickening of the wall prolongs the activation of the ventricle and as a result, the duration of the QRS complex. ST segment changes can also be present because repolarisation starts in the sub-endocardium instead of the sub-epicardium, or because permanent ischemia is present due to the increased left ventricular mass and reduced coronary blood flow. Typically the ST and T wave vectors have an opposite direction to that of the QRS complex. Electrocardiographic changes of right ventricular hypertrophy are seen only with severe right ventricular hypertrophy. The right electrical forces dominate the left electrical forces. Anterior forces will predominate with a tall R wave in V1 and a small S wave. In some cases the forces are posteriorly directed without changes in V1 but with a deep S wave in the left precordial leads. As with left ventricular hypertrophy, repolarisation is significantly modified with the vector of the QRS complex having an opposite direction to the vector of the ST segment (ST segment depression, T wave inversion in the right precordial leads). Left atrial enlargement prolongs the terminal portion of the P wave with an increased duration and a "double hump" or m-shaped morphology. Right atrial enlargement prolongs the initial portion of the P wave with a superimposition of its activation on the activation of the left atrium. As a consequence, the amplitude of the P wave increases in a triangular form without increasing its duration. Depolarisation of the atrium is best seen in leads II and V1. Enlargement of both atria is present when the criteria for both right and left atrial enlargement are fulfilled on the same ECG.

Keywords: Atrial hypertrophy, ventricular hypertrophy, QRS amplitude, P wave prolongation, P wave amplitude, bi-atrial hypertrophy, bi-ventricular hypertrophy, QRS axis, P wave axis.

LEFT VENTRICULAR HYPERTROPHY

Hypertrophy of the left ventricle causes a significant increase in the height and depth of the QRS complex. The thickening of the wall prolongs the activation of the ventricle and as a result, the duration of the QRS complex. ST segment changes can also be present because repolarisation starts in the sub-endocardium instead of the sub-epicardium, or because permanent ischemia is present due to the increased left ventricular mass and reduced coronary blood flow. Typically, the ST and T wave vectors have an opposite direction to that of the QRS complex (Figs. **1** and **2**) [1, 2].

Jean-Jacques Goy, Jean-Christophe Stauffer, Jürg Schlaepfer and Pierre Christeler

Diagnostic Criteria

Several criteria exist [1, 3].

The most common are the Sokolow criteria applicable when the duration of the QRS complex is < 120 ms.

Precordial leads:

S wave in V1 + R wave in V5 or V6 > 35 mm (Sokolow).

Tallest R wave + tallest S wave > 45 mm.

R wave in V5 or V6 > 26 mm.

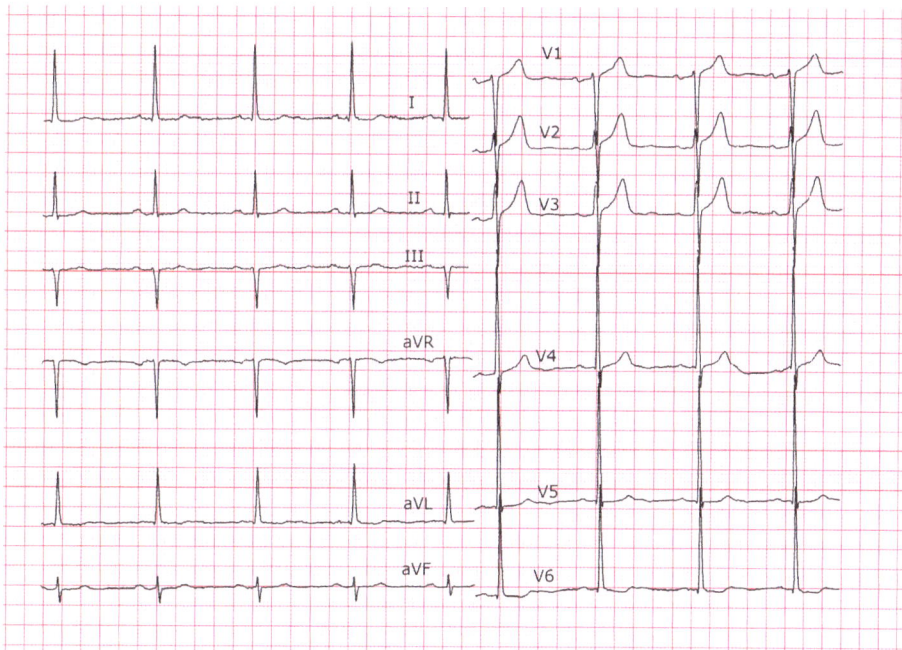

Figure 1: Left ventricular hypertrophy with multiple criteria present.

In the limb leads alone or in addition to the precordial leads:

R wave in I + S wave in III > 25mm.

R wave in aVL > 11mm.

R wave in aVL + S wave in V3 > 28 mm for females and > 20 mm for males.

Additional Criteria

The intrinsicoid deflection in V5 or V6 equal to or superior to 50 ms with ST segment depression, or T wave inversion in the left precordial leads or limb leads with a positive QRS complex. Generally, the sensitivity of these criteria varies between 25 and 50 %, and specificity is of the order of 90%. These criteria can only be applied to patients aged over 40 [2].

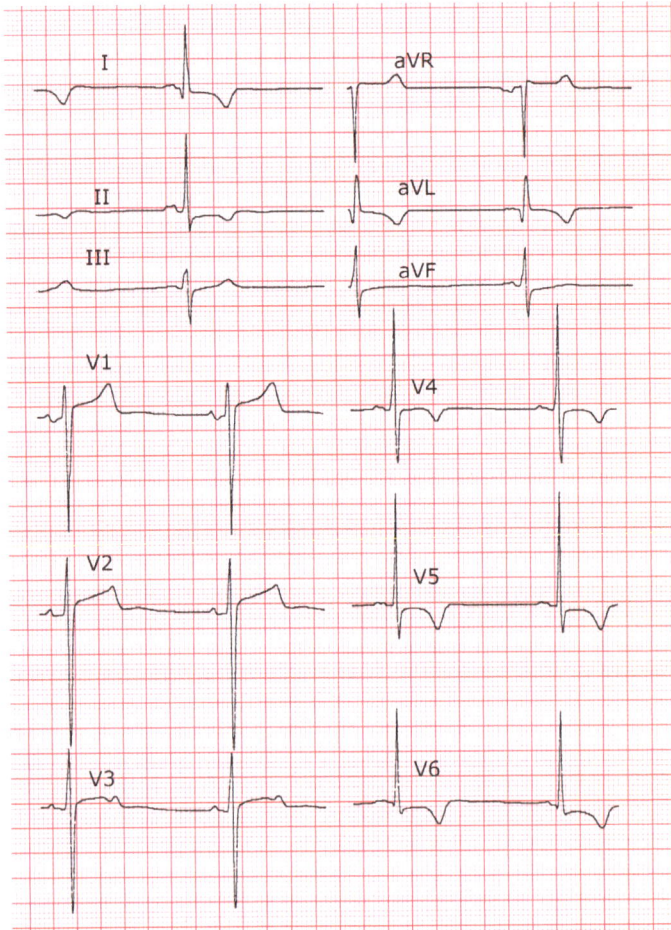

Figure 2: Left ventricular hypertrophy mainly visible in the left precordial leads (negative T waves in I, aVL, V4, V5 and V6). This trace is atypical for a true left ventricular hypertrophy. However, it is typical of hypertrophic obstructive cardiomyopathy (HOCM).

RIGHT VENTRICULAR HYPERTROPHY

The contribution of the right ventricle to the morphology of the QRS complex is almost non significant on the normal ECG. Thus, electrocardiographic changes are seen only with severe right ventricular hypertrophy. The right electrical forces dominate the left electrical forces. Anterior forces will predominate with a tall R wave in V1 and a small S wave. In some cases the forces are posteriorly directed without changes in V1 but with a deep S wave in the left precordial leads. As with left ventricular hypertrophy, repolarisation is significantly modified with the vector of the QRS complex having an opposite direction to the vector of the ST segment (ST segment depression, T wave inversion in the right precordial leads) (Fig. **3**). Sensitivity of these criteria is between 10 and 20%, even lower than those for left ventricular hypertrophy [1]. Specificity is around 90%.

Diagnostic Criteria

- They can be used only when QRS duration is < 120 ms.

- Right axis deviation $\geq 110°$.

- R/S in V1 > 1.

- R in V1, > 7mm.

- R in V1 + S in V5 or V6 > 10.5mm.

- R/S in V5 or V6 < 1.

- rSR' in V1 with R' $\geq$ 10mm.

HYPERTROPHY OF BOTH VENTRICLES

Diagnostic Criteria [4, 5-7]

- large biphasic QRS complexes in V2-5 (Katz-Wachtel phenomenon)

- S V2 + R V5 = 35 mm.

- R aVL > 11 mm with signs of LV strain (T-wave inversion in V4-6).

- Persistent S waves in V5-6 suggestive of associated right ventricular hypertrophy.

- S wave in V5-V6 > 7 mm.

- QRS amplitude > 50 mm in V2.

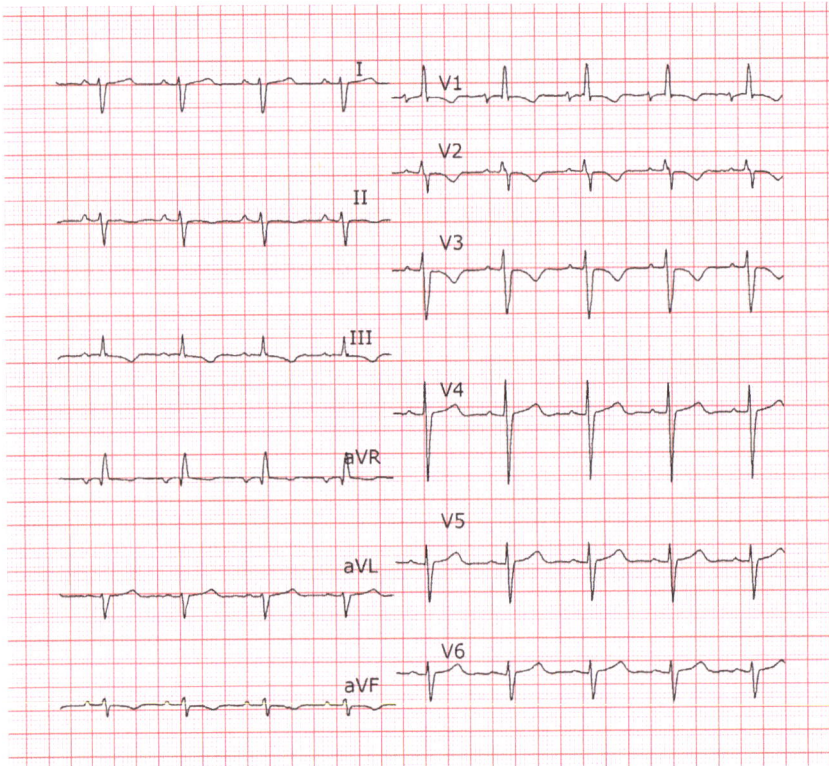

Figure 3: Right ventricular hypertrophy.

ATRIAL ENLARGEMENT

Left atrial enlargement prolongs the terminal portion of the P wave with an increased duration and a "double hump" or m-shaped morphology. Right atrial enlargement prolongs the initial portion of the P wave with a superimposition of its activation on the activation of the left atrium. As a consequence, the amplitude of the P wave increases in a triangular form without increasing its duration. Depolarisation of the atrium is best seen in leads II and V1 [8].

Diagnostic Criteria

Right atrial enlargement [1, 4] (Fig. **4**):

P wave amplitude > 2.5 mm in II.

Amplitude of the initial portion of the P wave > 1.5 mm in V1.

Frontal P wave axis ≥ 75°.

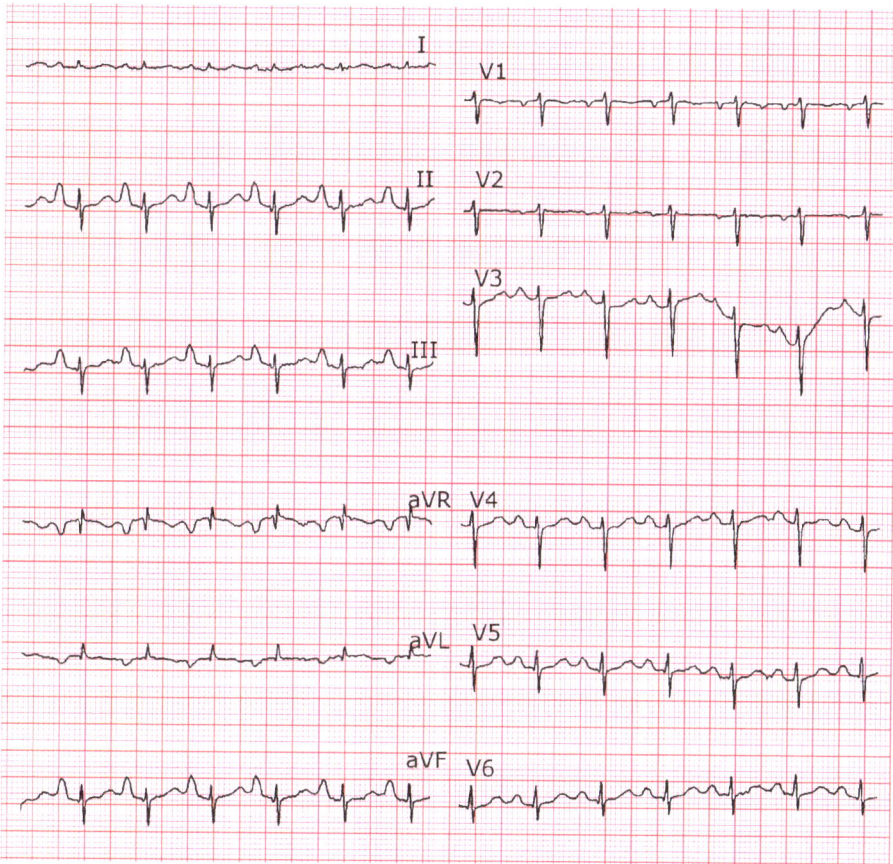

Figure 4: Right atrial enlargement.

Diagnostic Criteria

Left atrial enlargement [1,3] (Fig. **5**):

- P wave duration > 120 ms in II.

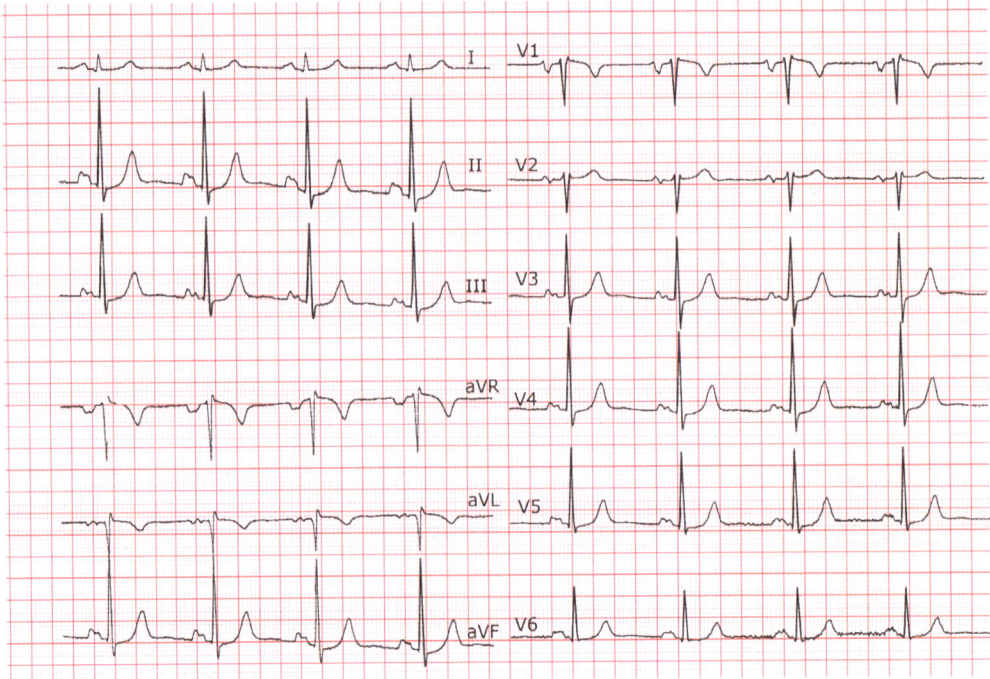

Figure 5: Left atrial enlargement.

-   In V1, prolongation of the final portion of the P wave (> 40 ms) and negative (> 1 mm).

-   Sensitivity of these criteria is low (approximately 10 to 20%) and specificity is around 80%.

ENLARGEMENT OF BOTH ATRIA

Enlargement of both atria is present when the criteria for both right and left atrial enlargement are fulfilled on the same ECG (Fig. **6**).

ACKNOWLEDGEMENT

Declared none.

CONFLICT OF INTEREST

The author(s) confirm that this chapter content has no conflict of interest.

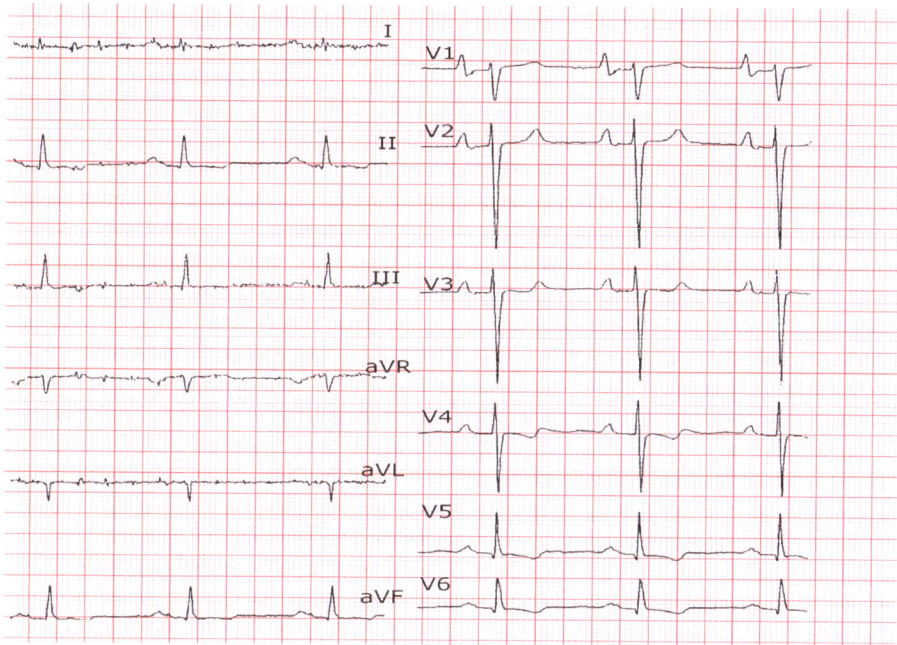

Figure 6: Enlargement of both atria with a combination of the criteria for left and right atrial enlargement.

REFERENCES

[1] Braunwald's Heart Disease : A Textbook of Cardiovascular Medicine: Elsevier- Saunders, 2011.

[2] Casale PN, Devereux RB, Kligfield P, *et al.* Electrocardiographic detection of left ventricular hypertrophy: Development and prospective validation of improved criteria. J Am Coll Cardiol 6:572-578, 1985.

[3] Hazen MS, Marwick TH, Underwood DA: Diagnostic accuracy of the resting electrocardiogram in detection and estimation of left atrial enlargement: An echocardiographic correlation in 551 patients. Am Heart J 79:819-828, 1997.

[4] Kaplan JD, Evans GT, Foster E, *et al.* Evaluation of electrocardiographic criteria for right atrial enlargement by quantitative two-dimensional echocardiography. J Am Coll Cardiol 23:747-752, 1994.

[5] Murphy ML, Thenabadu PN, de Soyza N, *et al.* Reevaluation of electrocardiographic criteria for left, right and combined cardiac ventricular hypertrophy. Am J Cardiol 53:1140-1147, 1984.

[6] Molloy TJ, Okin PM, Devereux RB, *et al.* Electrocardiographic detection of left ventricular hypertrophy by the simple QRS voltage-duration product. J Am Coll Cardiol 20:1180-1186, 1992.

[7] Jain A, Chandna H, Silber EN, *et al.* Electrocardiographic patterns of patients with echocardiographically determined biventricular hypertrophy. JElectrocardiol 32:269-273,1999.

[8]   Murphy ML, Thenabadu PN, de Soyza N, *et al.* Reevaluation of electrocardiographic criteria for left, right and combined cardiac ventricular hypertrophy. Am J Cardiol 53:1140-1147, 1984.

CHAPTER 8

Electrolyte Disturbances and QT Interval Abnormalities

Abstract: In this chapter, we address the basic notions of electrolytes disturbances and QT interval abnormalities. The most important abnormality of the QT interval is long QT syndrome, which provokes inhomogeneity of repolarisation with a marked tendency to induce severe ventricular arrhythmias (torsades de pointes). This long QT syndrome can be found in several clinical settings. The Jervell and Lange-Nielsen syndrome is an autosomal recessive form of long QT syndrome with associated congenital deafness and the Romano-Ward syndrome is an autosomal dominant form of long QT syndrome that is not associated with deafness. QT prolongation is associated with syncope (fainting) and sudden death due to ventricular arrhythmias (torsades de pointes). Arrhythmias are often associated with exercise or excitement. LQTS is associated with the rare, ventricular arrhythmia torsades de pointes, which can deteriorate into ventricular fibrillation and ultimately death. Several genetic mutations have been described. Syncope is usually the first manifestation of the syndrome. The acquired long QT syndrome is most often iatrogenic or associated with the following clinical situations: ischemia, subarachnoid hemorrhage, thyroid disease, electrolyte disturbances (hypocalcemia), side effects of drugs like antiarrhythmic agents (class IA, like quinidine, or class III like sotalol or amiodarone), antidepressant agents, some antihistamine drugs or even some other substances. Short congenital QT syndrome is a newly described disease characterized by a shortened QT interval, QTc, < 340 ms associated with episodes of syncope, paroxysmal atrial fibrillation or life-threatening cardiac arrhythmias. Hyperkalemia is the most dramatic and life-threatening electrolyte disorder. There appears to be a direct effect of elevated potassium on some of the potassium channels by increasing their activity and speeding up membrane repolarisation. Also, hyperkalemia causes an overall membrane depolarisation that inactivates sodium channels. The faster repolarisation of the cardiac action potential causes tenting of the T waves, and the inactivation of sodium channels causes sluggish cardiac conduction, which leads to smaller P waves and widening of the QRS complex. Hypokalemia Electrocardiographic findings associated with Hypokalemia are flattened T waves, ST segment depression and prolongation of the QT interval. U wave amplitude is slightly increased. It is rarely associated with arrhythmia. Hypercalcemia is associated with a shortening of the ST segment and consequently the QT interval. A very high Ca level broadens the T wave and may normalize the QT interval. Hypocalcemia prolongs the ST segment and the QT interval. Many drugs, especially antiarrhythmic drugs, can be implicated in QT interval prolongation. Class 1a antiarrhythmics significantly prolong the QT interval and may be responsible for ventricular arrhythmias like ``torsades de pointes''. Class 1c, mainly flecainide broadens the QRS complex by slowing conduction in the Purkinje fibres. Antidepressants may be responsible for severe arrhythmias and conduction abnormalities. Common adverse effects of digoxin include severe arrhythmias like ventricular tachycardia (fascicular origin). Conduction abnormalities and atrial tachycardia are also observed. The combination of increased (atrial) arrhythmogenesis and inhibited A-V conduction (like

Jean-Jacques Goy, Jean-Christophe Stauffer, Jürg Schlaepfer and Pierre Christeler

atrial tachycardia with A-V block) is said to be pathognomonic of digoxin toxicity, like fascicular ventricular tachycardia.

Keywords: QT interval, QT interval prolongation, hyperkalemia, hypokalemia, hypercalcemia, hypocalcemia, electrolytes disturbances, long QT syndrome, short QT syndrome, hypothermia, bidirectionnal tachycardia.

QT INTERVAL ABNORMALITIES

The most important abnormality of the QT interval is long QT syndrome, which provokes inhomogeneity of repolarisation with a marked tendency to induce severe ventricular arrhythmias (torsades de pointes) [1]. This long QT syndrome can be found in several clinical settings:

A) Congenital Long QT Syndrome

The Jervell and Lange-Nielsen syndrome is an autosomal recessive form of long QT syndrome with associated congenital deafness and the Romano-Ward syndrome is an autosomal dominant form of long QT syndrome that is not associated with deafness. QT prolongation is associated with syncope (fainting) and sudden death due to ventricular arrhythmias (torsades de pointes). Arrhythmias are often associated with exercise or excitement. LQTS is associated with the rare, ventricular arrhythmia torsades de pointes, which can deteriorate into ventricular fibrillation and ultimately death. Several genetic mutations have been described. Syncope is usually the first manifestation of the syndrome. In general, syncope requires a complete set of investigations when associated with stress or effort in young children or teenagers [7] (Fig. **1**).

B) Acquired Long QT Syndrome

The acquired long QT syndrome is most often iatrogenic or associated with the following clinical situations [7]. (Figs. **2** and **3**):

1. Ischemia.

2. Subarachnoid hemorrhage. (Fig. **2**) [2,3].

3. Thyroid disease.

4.   Electrolyte disturbances (hypocalcemia).

5.   Side effects of drugs like antiarrhythmic agents (class IA, like quinidine, or class III like sotalol or amiodarone), antidepressant agents, some antihistamine drugs or even some other substances. Exhaustive lists are available in the literature.

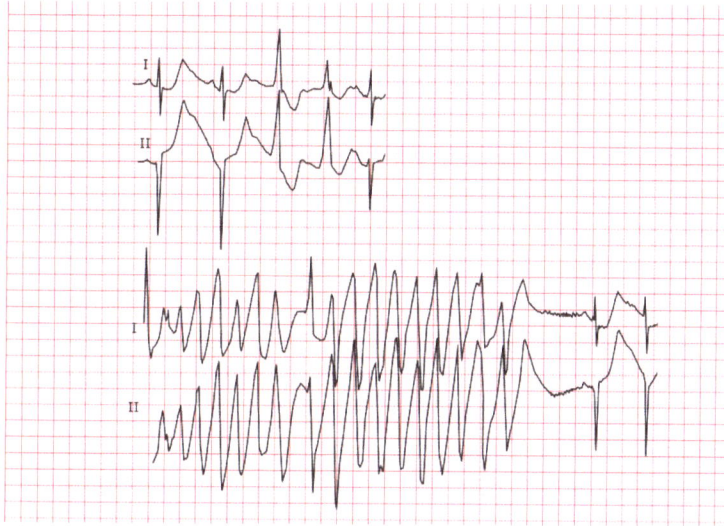

Figure 1: This trace shows sinus rhythm for the first 2 complexes with a markedly prolonged QT interval followed by the typical ventricular arrhythmia called "torsades de pointes". This is a case of congenital long QT syndrome.

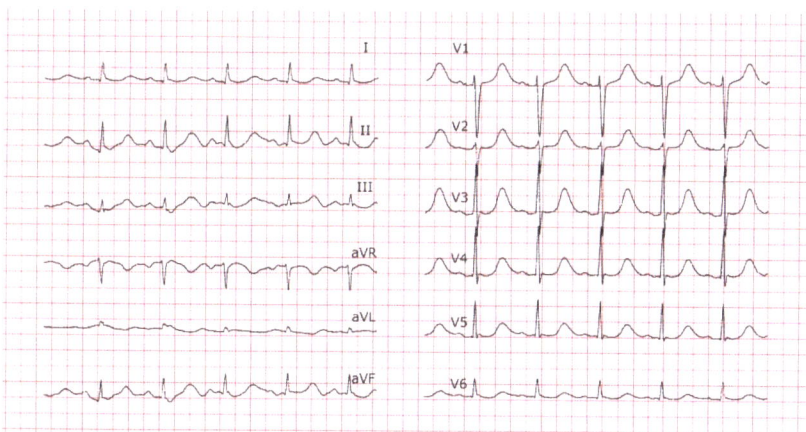

Figure 2: Prolonged PR interval at 220 ms. Massive QT prolongation at almost 600 ms due to a subarachnoid hemorrhage. Ventricular arrhythmias are almost inevitable with such QT prolongation.

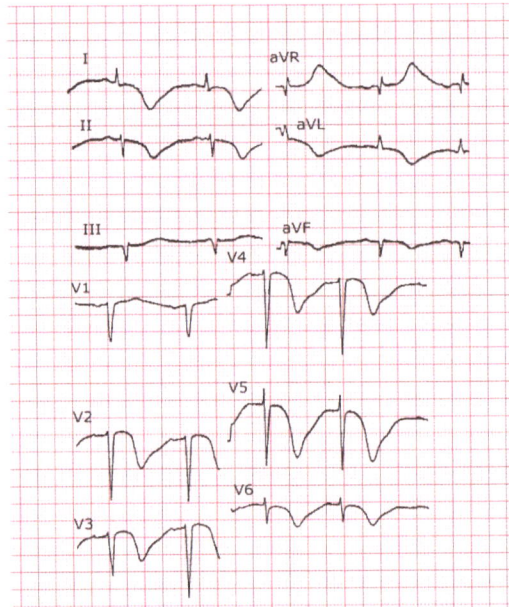

Figure 3: Regular sinus rhythm. "Grotesque" prolongation of the QT interval with deep and negative T waves due to quinidine treatment.

Short QT Syndrome

Short congenital QT syndrome is a newly described disease characterized by a shortened QT interval, QTc, < 340 ms associated with episodes of syncope, paroxysmal atrial fibrillation or life-threatening cardiac arrhythmias. Several genes have been described which cause mutations of potassium channels, leading to a shortening of the action potential. Sudden death has been reported with this syndrome. As the QT interval is only sligthly modified at high heart rates, the diagnosis is difficult especially in children. The T wave is tall and peaked. PR segment depression is sometimes present. During electrophysiological testing, ventricular fibrillation is easily inducible because of the short refractory periods (Fig. **4**).

ELECTROLYTE DISORDER

Hyperkalemia

It is the most dramatic and life-threatening electrolyte disorder. There appears to be a direct effect of elevated potassium on some of the potassium channels by increasing their activity and speeding up membrane repolarisation. Also, hyperkalemia causes an overall membrane depolarisation that inactivates sodium channels. The faster repolarisation of the cardiac action potential causes tenting of the T waves, and the inactivation of sodium channels causes sluggish cardiac conduction, which leads to smaller P waves and widening of the QRS complex [5-7].

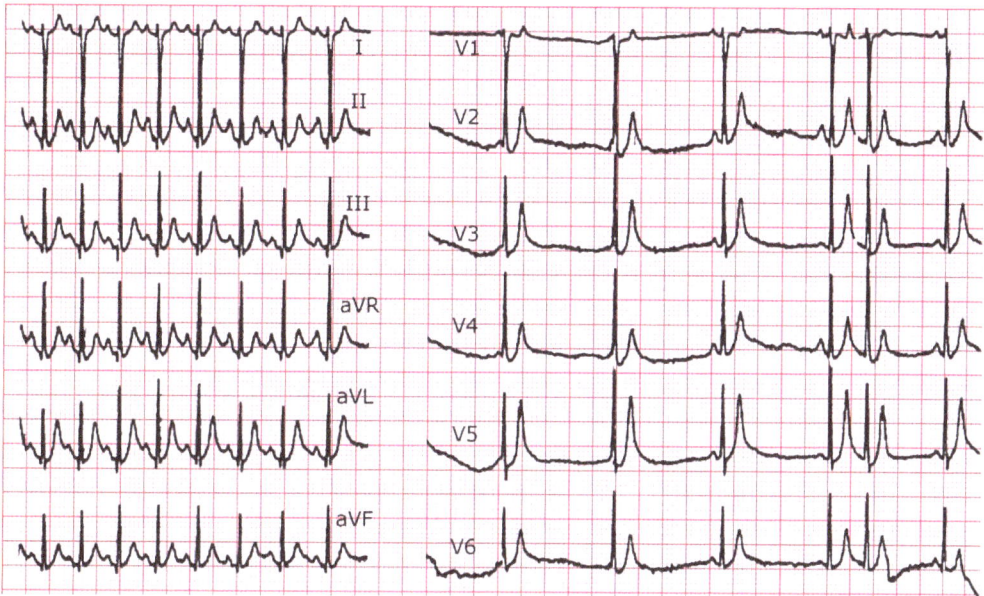

Figrue 4: Sinus rhythm on the left part of the trace with a QT interval at 240 ms. Sinus arrest followed by emergence of a nodal rhythm on the rigth part of the trace.

The 4 steps of hyperkalemia:

1. Stage 1 (K < 6.5 mmol/l): narrow T waves, tented with higher amplitude (Fig. **5**).

2. Stage 2 (6.5 < K < 7.5 mmol/l): tall, tented T waves with small P waves. Prolongation of the PR interval.

3. Stage 3 (7.5 < K < 8.5 mmol/l): significant widening of the QRS complex with disappearence of the P wave. Very positive T waves.

4. Stade 4 (K > 8.5 mmol/l): no clear separation between the QRS complex and the T wave. Extreme bradycardia. This rhythm precedes a cardiac arrest (Fig. **6**).

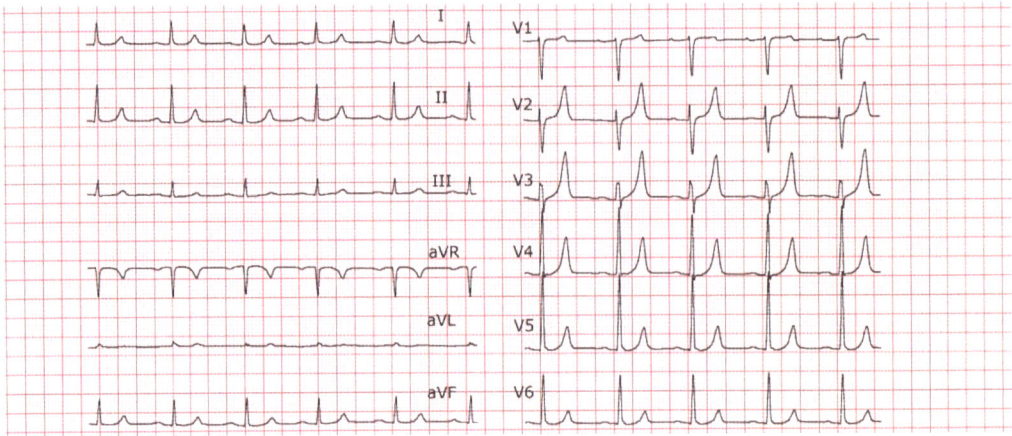

Figure 5: Sinus rhythm with almost invisible P waves. Tented T waves. hyperkalemia stage 2 (K = 7.1 mmol/l).

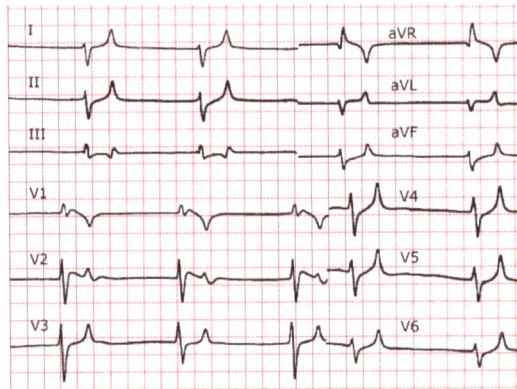

Figure 6: Idioventricular rhythm without P waves. Wide QRS complex with tented T waves and absence of clear separation between the QRS complex and the ST segment are prsent. Hyperkalemia stage 4 (K = 8.7 mmol/l).

Hypokalemia

Electrocardiographic (ECG) findings associated with hypokalemia are flattened T waves, ST segment depression and prolongation of the QT interval. U wave amplitude slightly increased. It is rarely associated with arrhythmia.

Hypercalcemia

Hypercalcemia is associated with a shortening of the ST segment and consequently the QT interval. A very high Ca level broadens the T wave and may normalize the QT interval [5].

Hypocalcemia

Hypocalcemia prolongs the ST segment and the QT interval [7].

Drug Related Abnormalities

Many drugs, especially antiarrhythmic drugs, can be implicated in QT interval prolongation. Class 1a antiarrhythmics significantly prolong the QT interval and may be responsible for ventricular arrhythmias like "torsades de pointes". Class 1c, mainly flecainide broaden the QRS complex by slowing conduction in the Purkinje fibres. Antidepressants may be responsible for severe arrhythmias and conduction abnormalities. Common adverse effects of digoxin include: loss of appetite, nausea, vomiting, diarrhea, blurred vision, visual disturbances (yellow-green halos, xanthopsia), confusion, drowsiness, dizziness, nightmares, agitation, and/or depression. Less frequent adverse side-effects include severe arrhythmias like ventricular tachycardia (fascicular origin) (Fig. **7**). Conduction abnormalities and atrial tachycardia are also observed. Digitalis decreases conduction of electrical impulses through the AV node and enhances automaticity. The combination of increased (atrial) arrhythmogenesis and inhibited A-V conduction (like atrial tachycardia with A-V block) is said to be pathognomonic of digoxin toxicity, like fascicular ventricular tachycardia.

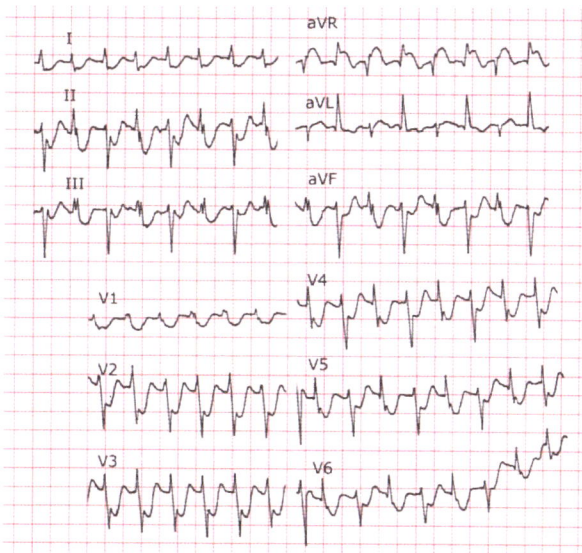

Figure 7: Bidirectional ventricular tachycardia as seen in digitalis intoxication.

In the clinical context, it should be borne in mind that antidepressant, antiarrhythmic, digitalis or any other medication can be associated with conduction abnormalities or severe arrhythmias.

Hypothermia

Hypothermia slows sinus activity and broadens the QRS complex. A positive deflection, Osborn wave, occurs at the junction between the QRS complex and the ST segment, the S point, also known as the J point (Fig. **8**) [7].

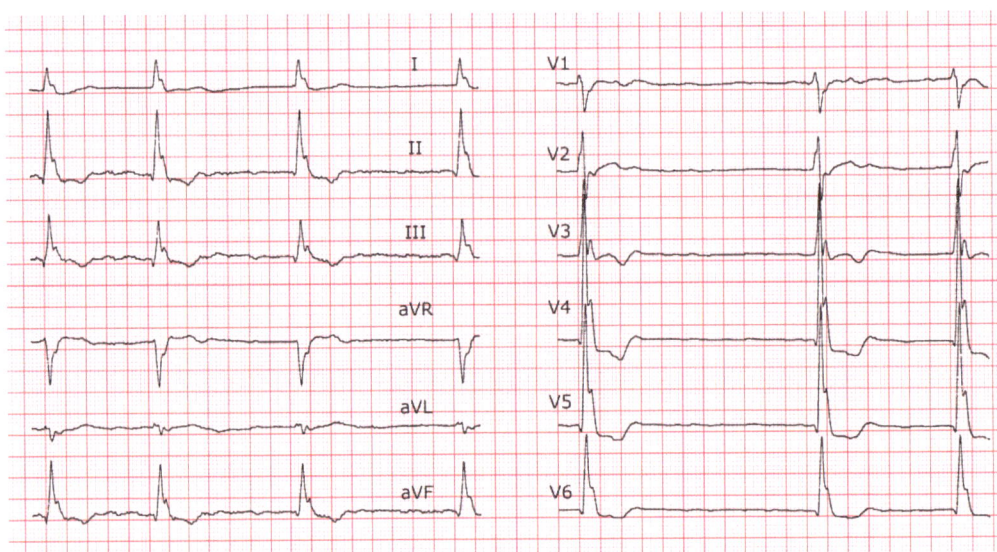

Figure 8: Slow atrial fibrillation with QRS widening as seen during hypothermia (Osborn waves).

ACKNOWLEDGEMENT

Declared none.

CONFLICT OF INTEREST

The author(s) confirm that this chapter content has no conflict of interest.

REFERENCES

[1]   Hingham PD, Campbell RWF: QT dispersion. Br Heart J 71:508, 1994.
[2]   Pollick C, Cujec B, Parker S, *et al.* Left ventricular wall motion abnormalities in subarachnoid hemorrhage: An echocardiographic study. J Am Coll Cardiol 12:600-605, 1988.

[3]   Elrifai AM, Bailes JE, Shih SR, *et al.* Characterization of the cardiac effects of acute subarachnoid hemorrhage in dogs. Stroke 27:737-741, 1996.

[4]   Reilly JG, Ayis SA, Ferrier IN, *et al.* QTc -interval abnormalities and psychotropic drug therapy in psychiatric patients. Lancet 355:1048-1052, 2000.

[5]   Ahmed R, Yano K, Mitsuoka T, *et al.* Changes in T wave morphology during hypercalcemia and its relation to the severity of hypercalcemia. J Electrocardiol 22:125-132, 1989.

[6]   Yu AS: Atypical electrocardiographic changes in severe hyperkalemia. Am J Cardiol 77:906-908, 1996.

[7]   MacFarlane PW, Lawrie TDV (eds): Comprehensive Electrocardiology: Theory and Practice in Health and Disease. Vol 3. New York, Pergamon, 1989.

INDEX

A

Aberrant conduction 57, 60, 63, 77-8, 84, 91-3

Abnormal depolarisations 56, 75

Accelerated idioventricular rhythm (AIVR) 96-7

Acquired long QT syndrome 98, 133-4

Activity 3, 10, 55, 133, 136

Acute coronary syndrome 100, 103

Acute pericarditis 116-18

Aid rhythm determination 23

Alternating atrial tachycardias 70

Antegrade conduction 54, 73-6, 78, 81, 87

Anterior infarcts 107, 109

Antiarrhythmic agents 133, 135

Antiarrhythmic drugs 67, 133, 139

Antidepressant 133, 139-40

Antidromic tachycardias 54, 78-9, 89, 92

Arrhythmia 6, 53-4, 57, 67, 70, 76, 80, 98, 116-17, 133, 138

Arrhythmogenesis 133, 139

Artery right coronary 100, 103, 109

Atrial arrhythmias 87

Atrial depolarization 4

Atrial extrasystoles 54

Atrial fibrillation (AF) 32-4, 53-4, 64, 67-71, 79-81, 87, 116-17

Atrial flutter 24, 32, 53, 65-7, 69, 83, 86, 92

Atrial hypertrophy 124

Atrial premature beats 53, 58-60

Atrial tachycardia 46, 54, 63, 65, 71, 76, 82-5, 133-4, 139

Atrio-ventricular block 27

Atrioventriuclar tachycardias 54

Atypical nodal tachycardia 83

Automatic tachycardias 70

AV nodal reentrant tachycardia (AVNRT) 53, 70, 76, 82-3, 85

www.ingramcontent.com/pod-product-compliance
Lightning Source LLC
Chambersburg PA
CBHW080020240326
41598CB00075B/599